# EACH Day ANEW

# EACH Day ANEW

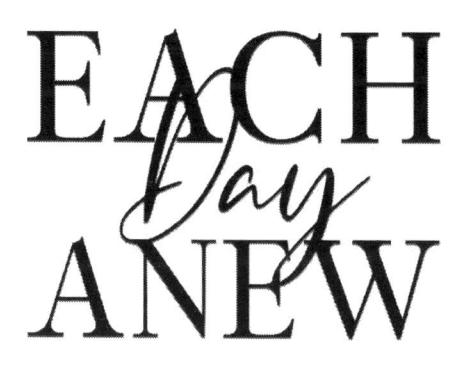

An Inspirational Autobiography

CANDY COCHRAN CRAIG

Copyright © 2022 Candy Cochran Craig
All rights reserved.
ISBN: 979-8-9862382-0-3

# DEDICATION

*Each Day Anew* is dedicated
to the memory of my mother,
with her amazing strength of character;
to my loving and devoted husband, Joel,
and to the praise and glory
of our Sovereign, Good and Loving God!

# CONTENTS

| | |
|---|---|
| INTRODUCTION | 1 |
| *Little Princess* | 5 |
| *Twists and Turns* | 15 |
| *Not "What" But "How"?* | 29 |
| *Not "Why" But "What Now"?* | 43 |
| *Live, Love and Learn* | 59 |
| *How Do You Feel?* | 85 |
| *Look Within: Time to Rest and Reflect* | 101 |
| *Look Up: For Rainbows and Silver Linings* | 113 |
| *Give It All You've Got And Go for It!* | 125 |
| *The End?* | 135 |
| ACKNOWLEDGEMENTS | 145 |
| A NOTE FROM THE AUTHOR | 149 |
| ABOUT THE AUTHOR | 151 |

# INTRODUCTION

For quite some time, I have wanted to write a book. I enjoyed creative writing as a child and was encouraged by one of my English teachers to submit essay and poetry selections to several publications. Throughout all my writings, whether poetry contests, school assignments or personal journal writing, I have found that expressing myself through words is very fulfilling. It has also become an effective tool for processing my life experiences and growing through the seasons of life. Seasons that included periods such as the turmoil of adolescence, the pursuit of education and career, as well as the joys and challenges associated with marriage and parenting.

Over the years, I have continued to think about writing a book and even talked about doing it. During certain periods of my life, I have been consistent about journaling my thoughts and feelings. With the onward march of time, I now find myself an empty nester, which provides a perfect opportunity to pursue this challenge and lifelong dream.

Whether we realize it or not, each of us is in the process of writing a book, and each day is a new page in our own personal story. My entire life is my book, filled with a variety of elements. These include such things as faith and circumstance, dreams and reality, joy and sorrow, acceptance and hope.

I find that I experience more enjoyable moments and successful outcomes in the various chapters of my life when I focus on maintaining a positive outlook. One way I do this is to consider each day like a new page in this book of life I am writing. The paper on which I write I call my opportunity to respond and the tools with which I write are the attitudes and beliefs that shape my responses to the happenings in my life. Although the topics are often chosen for me by the circumstances of each day, what I choose to write (how I respond) is always under my control.

Experiencing a lifelong chronic disease that has progressively limited my physical abilities and created a myriad of emotions has proved extremely challenging. It has been through the process of writing that I have been able to maintain a healthy balance in the way I respond to them. I have discovered that when I face *each day anew* then life becomes more bearable, more interesting, more purposeful, and even more enjoyable and hopeful! Some of these discoveries I plan to share with you in the pages ahead.

Perhaps you or someone you know yearns for a new beginning or a fresh start. My desire is to offer a way to approach life with optimism and hope. I want to encourage a life view that embraces life with all its ups and downs, twists and turns, periods of confusion and change as well as times of clarity, peace, and rest. As you read about some of my life's experiences and reflections, I hope you will become excited about your own stories and the book you are writing with your life.

I wrote the poem below over forty years ago which is still applicable today. It will give you an idea of the theme of this book. Give thought and consideration to how you, too, can approach each day as your "paper of opportunity" and then determine to begin "*each day anew*!

## EACH DAY ANEW

***GROW...***
Do not be afraid to reach upward toward tomorrow.
   Shed the leaves of yesterday.
   Do not be so rooted to the past
   that you do not continue
   to sprout forth and grow.
With the passing of each of life's seasons
   there can be painful changes
   and seemingly unending dormancy.
But take heart!
There is always the promise of another dawn,
   an awakening to the brilliant freshness
   of another day and a brand-new beginning!

***KNOW...***
That every day is like a blank tablet
   waiting to be written upon.
The pages of days gone by are yesterday's story.

Today begins a new page in your own book of life
   with great possibilities
   for enjoyment and adventure
   if not left on the shelf to collect dust.
Live out each daily scenario
   as if you are part of
   Life's number one best seller!

So, **GROW**
   in the knowledge
     as each day comes due,
and **KNOW**
   that by faith you can start
   **EACH DAY ANEW!**

*May you be rooted and established in love...*
*and grow in the grace and knowledge*
*of our Lord and Savior Jesus Christ.*
*Ephesians 3:18 and 2 Peter 3:18*
*(English Standard Version)*

# CHAPTER ONE
## *Little Princess*

I could think of no better way to begin my life story than to start at the beginning, and no better resource to consult than my mother. While reflecting with her upon my growing up years I became more aware of some of the factors that have shaped many of my attitudes toward life and the approach of starting *each day anew*. This first chapter will give you a glimpse of what it is like for a family who seems to be living life "happily ever after" to come to grips with the devastating effects of an unexpected diagnosis and learn to approach life with optimism and hope.

This chapter includes some of the reflections my mother shared with me, and by way of introducing myself, I share them with you. I am known to most everyone as "Candy" even though my name at birth was Candace. My petite stature has oftentimes given me a more youthful appearance than my actual age might indicate. As a teenager, I did not consider this an asset. However, my mother reassured me that one day I would appreciate my youthful appearance and that it would work to my advantage. I can honestly say that I have finally lived long enough to admit she was right.

I am a native Mississippian, born and reared in Jackson, the capital city. My parents grew up in rural southeast Mississippi. Having known each other in high school, they began dating afterward and married during World War II. My dad served in the Navy on a minesweeper in the Pacific. After the war, they moved to the Jackson area where they both attended Mississippi College. Upon completion of college, my father went to work for the Mississippi National Guard, and before long my older brother was born. Being the first grandchild on both sides of the family, his arrival warranted much attention and brought great joy and celebration.

The addition of a second child to our family did not occur as soon as they had hoped. Almost six years passed before my long-awaited arrival. The anticipation was great, especially for my brother, who was 5 ½ years old and eager for a baby sister. He planned to nickname me Candy. When an early false labor sent them back home from the hospital and my brother asked why he didn't have a baby sister yet, Daddy told him the hospital was just giving away boys so they would go back when they were giving away girls. A week later the hospital was giving away girls and I was born.

My mother reflects:

> Our beautiful little girl arrived in December, a dream come true to a loving and devoted mother, father, and little 5½ year old brother. What a happy and complete family we were with two beautiful and healthy children.

When I turned four, Mother returned to work as a legal secretary and employed our housekeeper, Helen, who became like a second mother to us and made it possible for us to stay at home instead of being placed in after school care. One of my earliest childhood memories is our move from a tiny two-bedroom house into a newer and larger ranch style three-bedroom home where I had my own room with *white princess furniture*.

We started out as a two-pet family. Ginger was a chihuahua that lived indoors and MiMi was a cocker spaniel who remained outdoors. One of my first exposures to loss was the death of Ginger after she was hit by a car. Daddy buried her in the backyard. The loss was offset greatly the following Christmas when our parents surprised us with a new poodle puppy that we named Bonnie Belle. Later, one of her puppies, Sugarfoot, was added to our family. All three dogs lived out long lives and brought us a great deal of happiness

My brother and I made friends readily in our new neighborhood. Our yard was often the gathering place for kickball games and ping-pong tournaments. Our old oak tree out back was home to a tree house constructed by Daddy and my brother, and it came fully equipped with a rope swing. Our fun in the tree house ranged from playing Tarzan to imagining ourselves as the Swiss Family Robinson.

My best friend lived in the house behind us. We were always together, either at my house or hers, so much so that Daddy cut an opening in the hedge of our backyard, and her father put a gate in their chain link fence just so we wouldn't have to walk along the street to get back and forth. She was the sister I always wished for, and to this day every time we talk or see each other we can pick up right where we last left off. My mother even fondly referred to her as "Daughter Number Two."

Our weekends and summer vacations became very treasured times for our family since both my parents worked full-time. Family vacations were always the last week of the summer before school started the day after Labor Day. They included one or two-week adventures to fun places like the Smoky Mountains in Tennessee, Pikes Peak in Colorado, or Disneyland in California. We usually went by car except for our first airplane trip to visit my cousin and her family in California. I remember marveling that they had an orange tree in their backyard from which my uncle would pick oranges and squeeze fresh orange juice every day for breakfast. Store bought juice was never the same after that.

I also have many fond memories of spending time at my grandparents' old country homestead in southeast Mississippi out in what we called "the middle of nowhere." It was especially great fun at family reunion time around the Fourth of July when as many as possible of my daddy's five siblings and their families would come.

There was always a big fish fry on Friday night made possible by multiple fishing trips by my aunt and uncle months prior to the reunion. Then on Saturday there would be a feast that put any Thanksgiving spread to shame. All the kids would circle around Granddaddy as he peeled fresh peaches, carefully peeling them so the peeling was an unbroken spiral that dropped into a scrap pail. Then he would cut a wedge of peach and drop it into the open mouths of grandchildren eagerly waiting for their turn, like baby birds as they anticipate the momma bird appearing with something good to eat.

Play time outside at Grandma's house was a great treat, especially for us city kids, as we got to go barefoot and climb the mimosa tree out front, despite many warnings to be careful. Visits in the summer months always included a swim in the bone-chilling creek, but only after the mandatory rest time to allow our dinner to settle. Many of us kids would wait eagerly for our turn in one of the rockers on the screened front porch or better yet, to be the victor in being the first one to claim the treasured porch swing. Finally, we would hear the awaited call for "swim time" and the race was on to see who could get their swimsuit on the fastest and be ready for the hike down to the creek. This was such a welcome treat during the heat of the afternoon and was intended for all ages.

Independence Day celebrations would end with going out to the field to watch fireworks, having the kids always sitting a safe distance away until it was time to end the display with sparklers. The girls imagined they were majorettes twirling fire batons while the guys had imaginary sword fights. We ended with one final parade in the dark before the sparklers went out. What fond and lasting memories!

Granddaddy was a Baptist circuit preacher and had a strong influence on our family. Rarely did we miss attending church, especially when we were at their house for a visit. We would always dress up in our Sunday best, which was usually what we had worn for Easter that year. I can still vividly picture their small un-airconditioned country church where we received cardboard fans stapled to popsicle sticks and sang old fashioned hymns making sure to sing all four verses.

Grandma was a bossy, but nurturing lady, who loved having crowds at her house. I remember her often saying, "there's always room for more!" She was the only person I knew who insisted on calling me Candace. I was told that she was the one who discovered the name Candace in the Bible and was influential in naming me. I also bear her middle name, Irene. To be honest, I much preferred the nickname Candy, but was always prompt in responding to "Candace Irene" whenever Grandma called.

One of my most treasured family traditions that our family still practices today came at Mother's Day. Each relative who could make it to Grandma's house for this special occasion received a freshly cut rose right out of her cherished rose garden to wear to church that day. It amazed me how Grandma's rose bushes were always blooming on Mother's Day weekend and there were always enough rosebuds to go around. You would get a red rose if your mother was living and a white one if she was deceased. From an early age, I remember being sad for my mother who always wore a white rose, because when she was 21, she lost her mother who died in a house fire. To this day, on every Mother's Day, I recall the many Mother's Days that God gave me with my mother, as she lived to be 93.

These and so many other events in my early years contributed to a happy and secure environment in which this "*dark haired little princess*" was treated like royalty, much loved and warmly nurtured.

Then, in the Fall of 1962, just prior to my sixth birthday, our lives were grievously interrupted by the onset of a sudden and severe illness. High fever, unexplained rashes and extreme pain in my hip prevented me from walking. I spent many weeks in the hospital undergoing a myriad of diagnostic tests. Life-threatening diseases such as leukemia were ruled out, and no stone was left unturned in the search for the problem underlying my puzzling symptoms.

After weeks with no answers, the pediatrician called Mother and Daddy to his office for a private consultation. They knew this was going to be profoundly serious news. Praying for strength before they left for the appointment better prepared them for the blow that came. Mother recalls their initial reaction:

> Our precious little girl had been diagnosed with Still's disease, otherwise known as Juvenile Rheumatoid Arthritis. Needless to say, we were devastated, but from the very beginning we determined to be positive and hopeful and keep leading as normal and happy a home life as possible.

My Parents had never heard of Still's disease, but my pediatrician educated them as best he could. They gathered and read all the material they could find on the subject. Bed rest and aspirin were prescribed and lots of tender loving care. My Great-Grandma Riley came to be with us that winter, and many quiet time activities were planned to keep me busy. My brother, a teenager by this time, was made fully aware of my illness. I adored my older brother and sensed in return, only love and concern with never any jealousy or resentment. I continued to live the life of *"daddy's little princess"* - just with an extra set of challenges.

***"Children are a blessing and a gift
from the Lord."
Psalm 127:3
(Contemporary English Version)***

# CHAPTER TWO
## *Twists and Turns*

A special poem that has brought me encouragement over the years is entitled "*Don't Quit,*" by Frank Stanton. It hung on Daddy's office wall and years after his death I discovered it in his belongings. It was printed on faded parchment, so I preserved it on a plaque, and it has hung in a prominent place in my home wherever I have lived over the past forty years. This poem in its entirety can be found in a later chapter. One of the phrases in the poem reads "Life is filled with its twists and turns as every one of us sometimes learns . . ." The diagnosis of Juvenile Rheumatoid Arthritis (JRA) certainly was a twist and turn in the life of our family. Mother and Daddy knew from the start that they would be rearing a child with incredibly special needs.

Many different kinds of twists and turns occur along the journey of living with a chronic inflammatory disease. My parents followed the doctor's instructions without hesitation. However, worsening of the disease with painful, swollen joints known as flares would be interspersed with relief of symptoms that were only temporary remissions. This roller-coaster pattern of changes in symptoms led my parents to become acutely aware of the special emotional needs that accompany such an unpredictable childhood illness.

I would experience periods of frustration and anger when I didn't fully understand why I had to take daily rests when other kids could remain outside and play. Fear and anxiety would creep in when multiple doctor visits required needle sticks, and I soon felt like a human pincushion. Loneliness and alienation occurred when I had to be exempt from physical education and couldn't try out for elementary cheerleader. Disappointment also came when I couldn't participate in the school marching band - something to which I had aspired, so as to follow in my brother's footsteps.

Another special challenge for my parents, due to the physical limitations caused by the disease, was to plan things for me to do that directed my energies and interests more toward mental activities rather than physical ones. I believe this is one of the wise things my parents did that prevented me from feeling "handicapped." Another positive outcome that resulted from the need for less strenuous activity was that I learned to read at an early age and loved it. I am convinced this nurtured my interest in creative writing and journalism. That, in turn, led me to submit work in essay contests, compose poetry, and eventually become editor of my high school newspaper.

In addition to reading, I had the opportunity to learn a variety of arts and crafts and was always working on some kind of new project. Not only were these hobbies fun, but they became a great benefit later in life when I began pursuing a master's degree in Occupational Therapy. I was able to draw upon my previous experience and familiarity with a wide variety of crafts and activities and use them to help others once they encountered unexpected twists and turns in their lives that resulted in changes beyond their control.

As mentioned earlier, I admired my brother who played the clarinet and became band captain his senior year in the high school marching band. When the reality hit that my joints were not going to allow me to do likewise, my parents wisely re-directed my musical interest to participation in the church choir where I learned to sing harmony as an alto. I was also encouraged to play the piano, which was good exercise for my hands, but also a challenge during periods of inflammatory flares that caused pain and swelling in my wrists and hands. But amazingly, I continued playing the piano all the way from second grade through high school and was even able to perform in a senior recital.

Also, as long as I could tolerate it, I was able to take tap, ballet, and jazz dance lessons for several years, but eventually the classes became too strenuous on my joints. However, my interest and appreciation of dance remained, and most years I have been in the audience at *The Nutcracker* or at the dance recital of one of my friend's children. Looking back, I realize that persevering with playing the piano, in spite of the pain and difficulty experienced at times, is what helped preserve the dexterity in my hands and maintain range of motion in my fingers and wrists. Additionally, not giving in to fear of pain and inability kept me active longer, thus preventing early crippling deformities and postponing the need for joint replacement surgeries until my young adult years.

I can now see that by encouraging my creativity, and modeling the attitude that said, "Let's see what you CAN do rather than being afraid that you can't," my parents contributed to my developing a very healthy self-esteem and a positive outlook on life. They were also successful in providing outlets for those frustrating times when my body simply could not do the things I so desperately wanted to do, such as marching band and continuation of dance classes.

The physical, emotional, and mental challenges of dealing with JRA had a great spiritual impact on me. My life experiences, as well as my parents, taught me about the providence and goodness of the One and Only Living God who knew me and formed me in my mother's womb. From His Word I learned that I am fearfully and wonderfully made. (Psalm 139:14, KJV) and therefore I am not defined by my disease or its limitations.

Having a chronic disease at such a young age also brought about the realization that life's true meaning and fulfillment must extend beyond the physical. Being raised and nurtured to have faith in God Who created and sustains all life, was the foundation established for me by my parents. Certain teachers at school and leaders at church contributed to my growing understanding of sin, mercy, grace, and eternal life.

One Easter, during the preacher's sermon, I became keenly aware that my personal suffering paled in significance to the sacrifice, pain and suffering Jesus Christ endured for my salvation. It was on that Easter Sunday, at age ten, that I made a profession of faith in Christ as my Savior and Lord. Over the years, God's personal presence in my life through the indwelling of The Holy Spirit, and His intimate involvement in my life amidst the many challenges of battling arthritis and its effects, have been primary factors in an ever-increasing dependence on God's great faithfulness. And my *"each day anew"* outlook echoes what is proclaimed in The Bible, "His mercies are new every morning." (Lamentations 3:23 ESV)

A great test of our entire family's faith and dependence upon God came when I was age 12 and approaching adolescence. On Mother's Day, 1969, I suddenly began to vomit blood and was rushed to the hospital. I was bleeding internally, but initially the cause was unknown. We did not realize it at the time, but the medications prescribed for the control of my arthritis caused an ulcer in my stomach which was the size of a half dollar. It perforated my aorta, the largest artery of my body that carried blood from my heart to the rest of my body. As fast as I could receive blood transfusions, I was losing it through internal bleeding.

I required emergency surgery and 24 additional units of blood just to keep me alive. To make matters worse, in all the confusion with the exploratory surgery, one of the units of blood I received was the incorrect blood type, which we later learned had the potential to shut down my kidneys and send me into congestive heart failure. I spent several weeks in critical condition in intensive care with my family not knowing if I would live or die.

Once I was stable from the emergency surgery, other complications arose. I developed problems with my liver which resulted in jaundice. Additionally, the lining around my heart became inflamed causing chest pain. From

Mother's Day to Labor Day of 1969, I spent a total of 94 days in the hospital, which meant so did my parents, who took turns staying the night so I wouldn't be alone and would be sure to get the attentive care I needed.

After three months of hospitalization, we were hopeful the worst was behind us, but it was not the case. The aftermath of the fierce battles my body had undergone, as well as my inability to tolerate the medications I needed for treatment of my arthritis, caused the disease to rear its ugly head and the flares of inflammation, pain and swelling became worse than ever. The disease had exceeded the expertise of my pediatrician, so I was referred to a rheumatologist who was an arthritis specialist. Much to my despair and that of my parents, it became necessary for me to be placed in an inpatient rehabilitation institution where my medical, therapeutic, and educational needs could be met. When I was admitted, my prognosis was uncertain, and the length of stay was considered indefinite. It was my plan, however, to spend as little time there as possible and I was determined to shorten the doctor's projected stay of an entire school year to just one semester. I entered in August and was home by Christmas, certainly something unexpected by my doctor's standard.

It was during this time that my entire family and I experienced some of our darkest days. Unfortunately, my health complications came at a time when my brother was the first birdie to leave the nest, initially for college and, soon thereafter, military service during the Vietnam War. Mother told of many days when she would arrive home from work and find Daddy sitting alone on our patio, still in his military work uniform, unable to enter the unbearably lonely house. It had become more than simply empty; it was completely void of the boisterous activity of his teenage son who now faced the rigors of war and the unknown outcome of a safe and sound return. Gone also was the cheerful greeting from his "sweet little princess" who was facing grave uncertainty from a potentially crippling disease.

It was a sorrowful time for all of us. However, in the midst of our suffering, God demonstrated His great faithfulness to us, not only by sparing my life from a near death experience, but also daily sustaining us through some of the devastating effects of living with a childhood chronic disease.

After months of separation from my parents due to the time spent at the rehabilitation institute, I returned home and began the uphill climb of learning how to live life daily and deliberately, with the unpredictable nature of a disease that was taking quite a toll on my life. My first weeks of adjusting to the rigorous schedule of junior high school were met with exhaustion and tears. Having to climb stairs to reach certain classes before the class bell rang often resulted not only in physical pain but in fear of tardiness and embarrassment.

It was during these years that God transformed my feelings of anger, resentment, and fear into the positive character traits of perseverance, patience, and determination. These traits came to shape my outlook on life and enabled me to cope successfully in the days and years ahead.

Following three years in junior high school, interspersed with joint repair surgeries and physical therapy during the summers, I was more than ready to begin the excitement of high school. I became interested in journalism and drama and was actively involved in extracurricular activities such as our high school newspaper and several school musicals. It was interesting to find out at our first high school reunion, after I had been away to college and undergone several joint replacement surgeries, that many of my high school classmates shared that they never realized that I had arthritis or that there was anything wrong with my health.

This speaks highly of the atmosphere and attitude of "normalcy" that my parents so diligently tried to achieve in our family. They worked hard to maintain a healthy balance between proper management of the disease without letting it consume our lives. However, as I discovered when talking with my mother, it did not come without struggles on their part. Mother confided:

> Rarely would Candy say "no" to anything she was asked to do. I often conferred with her doctor as to how we could say no to things we knew might be too much for her. His advice was, "Let her lead with her own head and her own heart, and she will soon learn for herself what and how much she can handle."

By my parents following this advice, sometimes I paid the cost for overdoing it. Sometimes it was worth the effort that it took and the consequences that followed. Overall, I learned many life lessons and was the wiser for it. I'm grateful for how my parents fostered my independence.

Mother also recalled a difficult decision she and Daddy had to make regarding allowing me to spread my wings, and them resisting the tendency to be overprotective. She shared:

> One event that really tested our letting Candy exercise her independence was when she wanted to take a trip abroad with her high school Latin class. We knew this would be a huge test for her, being far away from home and having to pace her daily activities as determined by her health. However, we knew this experience would increase her confidence and her aspirations for higher education and future endeavors. Reluctantly we agreed for her to go. Our hearts ached each day she was away, and we rejoiced when she returned, and everything had gone well. We were convinced then that Candy would

accomplish whatever she set her mind to do, and we resolved to give her all the opportunities, encouragement, and educational advantages we could afford.

Another devastating *twist and turn* in our lives came the summer between my junior and senior years in high school. Daddy experienced a sudden and fatal heart attack at age fifty. He had just been to National Guard summer camp at Camp Shelby and passed his physical with flying colors. With the exception of a long-standing stomach ulcer caused by stress and having the middle-age spread we kiddingly called a pot belly; Daddy was in good health. But one night just prior to bed he had what he thought was his usual ulcer pain. When he sat up to go get his antacid medicine he just suddenly collapsed back onto the bed and died instantly. This was in 1974 prior to any of his other five siblings' deaths. Only years later was it discovered that aneurysms ran in the family. Three out of the remaining five siblings died suddenly or in their sleep with an aneurysm.

Daddy's unexpected death rocked our world in so many ways. Mother became a single parent and again worked hard to maintain a new normal in our lives. She strongly encouraged me to continue to participate in my extracurricular activities such as the school musical and editor of our school newspaper, even though both of these commitments required after school and late-night hours. Mother also insisted that I continue with my plans to go away to college instead of remaining at home and attending a local one. She said Daddy had wanted to attend the college I had chosen but had to go where his parents suggested instead.

Years later, Mother reflected how glad she was that she and Daddy had decided to go ahead and allow me to travel to Italy at the end of my sophomore year instead of waiting until the following year. so he could see the joy and self-sufficiency it brought me. Also, Mother confessed how hard she had lobbied with Daddy for me to receive my own car for my 17th birthday instead of waiting until I turned 18. We still have the video of my red, white, and blue bicentennial 1976 Chevrolet Vega hatchback sitting in the driveway with a huge red bow across the windshield as I approached blindfolded. It was truly the surprise of my life. And of course, it had standard transmission since Daddy insisted that we first learn to drive a stick shift.

Mother summarized her philosophy in parenting a child with a chronic disease, both with Daddy and alone after he died, by emphasizing her dependence upon God for patience, perseverance, and wisdom. Mother often wondered if God took Daddy early, before all my replacement surgeries began, because it pained him so for me to be in the hospital and suffer pain.

Mother is the one who would remind me never to say or even think, "*I can't*," instead she encouraged me to say, "*I will try*." I also learned it was perfectly normal to ask "*Why?*" or wonder "*Why me?*" I also saw how my parents moved beyond the "*why*" to the "*what do we do now*?" These attitudes had a tremendous influence upon how I came to approach *each day anew*. In retrospect, Mother affirmed:

> Despite many painful and difficult moments throughout our lives, my prayers for our *precious little princess* have been answered and my dreams have come true. See for yourself as she shares many of her life stories and life lessons with you. See how God has enabled one afflicted little girl to approach *each day anew*!

**"... we know that suffering produces perseverance; perseverance, character; and character, hope."**
**Romans 5:3b-4**
**(New International Version)**

# CHAPTER THREE
## Not "What" But "How"?

When I first decided I wanted to write a book (over 40 years ago) my initial question was not so much "what" but rather "how?" Do you sit down at a typewriter and type nonstop? Do you get a tape recorder and pour out your life story from day one? Just how do you do it? Well, an inquiry into the matter resulted in as many different answers as individuals that were asked.

But one suggestion impacted me more than all the others. It came from my Uncle Sam who was a most interesting character. He was the oldest of my daddy's siblings and over the years we heard snippets of his ventures as a World War II pilot. He was also an avid cyclist and even cycled across the country at the age of 70. He published a book about his cycling journey, and after his death we discovered stories that he had written about his WWII exploits. Uncle Sam was a regular letter writer and often sent copies of his letters (the carbon paper kind) to my mother which I found in her files. (She was a keeper of letters and cards.) The unusual part about his letters was that he just sent the first page, which often stopped in the middle of a sentence, and many times left you wanting more.

Another interesting thing was that Uncle Sam always had a journal with him (the gray hardback ledger kind). One year at our annual family reunion I asked him about his journal, his writings, and the book he published, and I shared with him that I was considering writing a book. He was all for it and I can still remember the way he enthusiastically clapped his hands together and said, "What a great idea!" When I asked him WHAT I should do he said "well, start with the HOW and just write!" He had an extra gray ledger with him that he gave me and told me to just start journaling.

He showed me his journal and I noticed that some of the entries were just a few words or sentences, while others were pages long. He said sometimes he wrote about feelings, other times about facts. He might just describe a flower he had seen that day or perhaps a memory from long ago. He told me that journaling would help me develop the habit of writing and give me practice in expressing myself. He suggested that I journal for a year and then look back over my entries and I would discover the "WHAT" that God had for me to share with others.

Well, the journal seemed like a good idea, so I decided to do just that. The first year I was not very disciplined about writing, so I actually ended up journaling for two years before I was able to look back and see a pattern and a life message emerging. Much of my first attempt at writing this book simply contained excerpts from my journal, as it is those day-to-day feelings, those ups and downs, that make up our lives. When I first sat down over 40 years ago to "write a book" this is what I began with:

> It's funny. I thought this would be the first page of my book. I guess I thought I would feel some sort of revelation or see stars or feel professional, but as I look closer, I find that this isn't really page one, for my whole life is my book. My life is what I want to share – through poems, prose, attitudes, beliefs & experiences. When you look at it from that point of view, this should not be such a hard job after all. So, what is holding me back? I think it has something to do with the same principle as that involving faith. You can say you believe in something, but not until you act on that belief, do you really exhibit faith. I believe I have something worthwhile to say. Sometimes I doubt myself and my capabilities. I think that at times we all do. Sometimes I fear failure. That fear paralyzes millions. But it is the ultimate belief that dreams can become realities which continues to drown out those doubts and fears and drive me onward. The time has come to put my faith into action, and in this case, it means putting my beliefs into words. Words that can speak in my absence; words that can convey meaning even after the initial thought or idea has passed on by. Words are a form of communication. They are symbols of meaning, that when combined in certain ways, convey a message. It is the message that is the

key point of any act of communication, whether verbal or nonverbal. I will be sharing with you many of my early journal entries and you will see, as I did, how my theme and message of "new beginnings" and being able to start *"each day anew"* just seemed to naturally unfold.

And yes, I still journal! I have boxes of my journals (mainly steno pads – not hardback gray ledgers) that perhaps will mean something to those who come after me . . . or not. So, without further delay, (since it has been over 40 years since that first effort) I invite you to journey with me, and walk through a variety of my life experiences, thoughts, and feelings, as I learned (and am still learning) step by step, and day by day that a meaningful life is not just a destination, but more of a process.

My first journaling efforts began with New Year's Day 1978. It seemed a good time to begin, because I had just received the first of my joint replacement surgeries in Fall 1977, bilateral total hip replacements, and I was headed back to college after what I felt had been a devastating interruption in my life. But God was providentially working to direct and re-direct my life. Journaling is just one way He would reveal His plans and purposes for me in the days ahead:

> January 1, 1978: I am going to attempt to convey some of my feelings and experiences in this journal. I want to relate to you, to whomever, and really to

myself, just what life is all about - its newness, its beginnings, its endings, its abundance. I hope it will lead to a book of my own. Tomorrow I will start anew. Until then I must rest. – Candy.

Well, "tomorrow" came several weeks later:

<u>January 17, 1978:</u> It is hard to believe that I have begun again. A logical place to start to tell a story would be at its beginning. It is this point which baffles me, for my life has been nothing but one new beginning after another. If there is one important idea that I can convey, it is the splendid fact that you can start "*each day anew*" learning from all your yesterdays and striving toward your tomorrows. It is today with which I will now begin. To explain my feelings today, I must refer to my yesterdays.

Four months ago, I was in pain, mentally, emotionally, and physically. I was about to undergo bilateral hip replacement surgery and I felt as if I was in a world of detachment and unreality. I was living on hope and faith that my "tomorrows" would somehow hold relief from all my "yesterdays of suffering." I am here today as a fulfillment of that hope and a result of God's faithfulness in my life. I am now facing reality with an awareness unlike ever before. I have begun again, and I am thankful for the experiences of today, the lessons of yesterday and the promises of tomorrow.

Then I did not write again until five months later and again it involved a "first":

<u>June 21, 1978:</u> Today is the first day of summer. Life is in its fullest array everywhere I look. And that includes my life. It has been five months, a whole semester, and a world of emotions and feelings ago since I last sat down to write. My yesterdays have no

longer been ones of pain and suffering but rather ones of fulfillment and growth. I have watched myself learn things all over again that I had known forever, but in the hustle and bustle of my everyday scramble, I had failed, to realize. Things such as what it felt like to experience a pain-free brisk walk to class on a cool spring morning or learning about problem-solving methods in theory and then actually applying them. Also getting to visit with an old acquaintance and listening -- really listening -- and giving support and guidance to a friend in need and reaping the satisfaction of her victory and success. Then there were the simple joys of giggling with my mom, watching my niece take those first few steps, and now I'm just sitting outside on this step sharing and caring about the little things in life that make it so abundant and worthwhile. I am firmly convinced that God is in complete control of my life. How else could I have been lifted from pain and suffering into a life abundant and fulfilling? Most importantly, there is a point I must make. My foundation to begin with is a firm one. It is Jesus Christ. It is through my faith in Him that all life experiences have been strengthening ones. As an illustration, let me include this poem by Jane Merchant that I memorized:

> *Full half a hundred times I've sobbed,*
> *"I can't go on; I can't go on"*
> *And yet full half a hundred times*
> *I've hushed those sobs and gone.*
> *The answer, if you ask me how,*
> *may seem presumptuously odd.*
> *But I know that what kept keeping on*
> *when I could not, was GOD!*

I know not what the future holds, but I know He holds the future! --until later, Candy

P.S. The chorus of one of my favorite southern gospel songs written by Ira Stanphill also reinforces this theme.

*Many things about tomorrow
I don't seem to understand
But I know God holds tomorrow and
I know He holds my hand!*

The previous entry was during the summer, the following one came during Fall:

<u>November 1, 1978:</u> Today was full of new life. Even though the fall season spells a natural "slow-down" of nature, new beginnings are still everyday occurrences. Today was the first day of a new month; I ate lunch with a new friend at an old boarding house to which I had never been. I saw a new-born baby. I greeted a newlywed couple just back from their honeymoon. I shared a vision with a friend to return to school – another new and exciting beginning in her life. Like the naked eye without the microscope, we oftentimes cannot see the teeming life so abundant in the pond. We are quick to notice the scum on top of the pond and make judgments according to the appearance of the surface but forget that it is the life beyond the "apparent" that gives sustenance to the whole. So, it is in everyday living. We take life so flippantly and at surface value. We are so quick to point out the scum and get so bogged down in the mud that we fail to look beyond to the abundance that exists in our lives, every moment of every day that we live. In that way every experience is full of new life - growing, maturing, and becoming -- a constant renewal -- a beginning again and again and again. We are not merely human "beings" rather we are human "becomings".

During my first year of attempting to journal, it seemed that writing just didn't flow like I thought it would. I managed to take time to record my inspirations only about every four to six months. Then in May of the following year, 1979, I seriously began writing every day. This is not to say that inspiration poured forth constantly, but rather my ambition and drive were stronger. Through the discipline of writing God was giving me a clearer perspective, as can be seen in the following passages:

> May 17, 1979: Today was a day of beginning again. Just about a year ago my whole life took on a new perspective. It all seems to be coming into focus slowly like a fog clearing into a bright fresh new morning. Often it is easier to see things clearer by going away and coming back, or even being apart from it for a while. Dormant periods, every now and then, are needed in order to appreciate the growing, productive, active times. I spoke with friends today about writing my very own book. Some look at me funny, others are encouraging, but it is the reality of my dream that I'm attempting to pursue, with the help of God - may it be done!

Over the course of journaling, I learned that times come in life when you cannot bring yourself to do something, even when you want to, or know you should. The act of writing is no exception. It's not always easy to write and express yourself. But it is during these times that attempts, despite lack of ability or desire, can be very revealing and even rewarding! A few examples follow:

August 11, 1979:  I so want to write or at least contribute in some way that would be worthwhile but for some reason I feel all clammed up. I feel like a bubble that is floating around and wants to land but is afraid if it stops or touches anything it will pop and disappear. I'm not sure how this analogy fits me, I'm just feeling weird these days. My body constantly reminds me that it is less than perfect. My mind constantly reminds me that I need to be doing something useful and productive with myself, and I'm having trouble with what God is telling me -- but then perhaps I'm not listening well.

These new beginnings in my life should be full of vigor and vitality and freshness, but instead I seem to be holding back. Perhaps I am afraid or hesitant to step out. But what I know to be true is that God wants what is best for me.  He leads me to and through endeavors in which I can express the best of who I am, who He has created me to be.  I can trust in His Spirit to lead, guide, direct and equip me.  If there seem to be walls around me that are way too high, then I can look for doors to open.

Heavenly Father, my prayer is that you will cleanse me of all unrighteousness, and as the old familiar hymn that I have heard innumerable times says,
   *Have Thine own way Lord,*
   *have Thine own way.*
   *Thou are the Potter; I am the clay.*
   *Mold me and make me, after Thy will.*
   *While I am waiting, yielded and still.*
   *(Lyrics by Pollard Stebbins)*
          Love, Candy

August 28, 1979: Today a chapter ends.  I will be heading out to Houston to begin another chapter in my book of life – graduate school!  May God continue to work in my life and in the lives of those

I encounter. This next year will bring about new horizons, intellectually, socially, emotionally, and even spiritually. Only God knows!

My move to Houston had its ups and downs. One day I felt like conquering the world and the next day, what a bummer. Once again, however, writing allowed me to come to grips with my feelings, acknowledge them, and process them.

> September 6, 1979: For some reason I have been hindered from writing the past month. Whether it has been a lack of time, motivation, or just plain fear, I'm not sure, but now is the time to begin again and that is the theme that seems to keep surfacing - NEW BEGINNINGS. The past month has been good. I feel fairly oriented to my new Houston environment for my occupational therapy graduate studies. I am living in the heart of the medical center, and I meet new people every day. A longtime friend who is also here in grad school has been helping me adjust. We have been making a point of getting out, meeting new friends, and having Christian fellowship. Classes are keeping me busy, in addition to other activities. I am finding the whole occupational therapy experience in the clinics to be very stimulating and challenging. However, other things confuse me if I let them. Missing my friends at home and concern for their well-being, wanting someone to share my life with, wanting to belong, particularly with a Christian fellowship, and trying to absorb all I can academically - all these things weigh me down sometimes. But I know this is where I should be. Working it all out is what life is all about.

## EACH DAY ANEW

The next day, September 7, 1979: Lord, I need peace like a river . . . so flow through me. Today has been a day of emotional strain. I worked with kids all day in kindergarten evaluations, so my patience was well tried. That, in addition to not feeling my best physically, has just about done me in. Life is trying here, but the promise of new beginnings sure does help. Anyway, I feel a freshening and a peace already beginning to flow. I talked to Mother today and the home front looks troubled. I must be sure to keep sending my support, in thoughts and prayers, as well as letters and calls. I really enjoyed the Bible study that I attended tonight. In it we explored incorporating spiritual care into health care. If we will simply build bridges to people through unconditional love, then Jesus can easily walk across. So much for sitting down to complain about my day. You see, just as a simple narrative can change moods midstream, so can life attitudes turn around. A "minus" (-) can become a "plus" (+) just by using one simple *cross*. Even more so the *Cross* of Christ can change any life for the better! (I enjoy using puns.) -- Candy

October 30, 1979: Today was a good day. I awoke ready to start it. I really like that refreshed feeling, a true answer to prayer.

November 1, 1979: Another beginning, another new month, and this one is gonna be super. Must rest for now. Life ahead looks good.

December 6, 1979: Well, I am surviving, and quite well at that! Another new beginning today -- my 23rd year! It has been a bit unusual, not your average celebration with cake and ice cream. The highlights have been in the little things -- a card, a happy birthday message on a blackboard, calls from my friends from afar, etc. I guess it's the little things that count the most in life anyway. Beginning another year in life has a way of giving us a new perspective, merely by being something new. The ending of one year and the beginning of another serve as a vantage point -- a point at which one can look backward and forward at the same time. CC

And the ending of the calendar year also brings reflections:

December 30, 1979: One more day in this year. The semester was good. I learned to listen more -- to myself, to others, and most importantly, to God. With the coming of the new year, I am anticipating further becoming what God wants me to be. I'm glad God is in the driver's seat of my life. Even though the road gets curvy or even treacherous at times, I know that He knows the final destination and will get me there safely. As He teaches me how to better navigate the various twists and turns of my life's path, I want to be an attentive learner. I know that He has and continues to teach me that His mercies are indeed new and abundant every morning, enabling me to begin *each day anew!*

In sharing with you my early journal entries and some of those that followed, perhaps you can see, that life itself writes its own book and the exercise of writing can be a great tool for personal reflection and growth. It gives us an opportunity to record and process facts, feelings, events, experiences, responses, relationships, obstacles, detours, dreams, failures, and victories – all a part of our life journey. It's not so much the "WHAT" in our journey - the accomplishments or the destinations - that count, rather it's more the "HOW" - the process of our own personal journey - that becomes more meaningful as we approach *each day anew*. With this assertion I shall continue to share with my life experiences, my journey, and how God has continued to reveal His great faithfulness and new mercies every morning!

> *"Because of the LORD's great love,*
> *we are not consumed,*
> *for His compassions never fail.*
> *They are new every morning.*
> *Great is Your faithfulness."*
> *Lamentations 3:22-23*
> *(New International Version)*

# CHAPTER FOUR
## Not "Why" But "What Now"?

Many folks dwell on the "whys" in life and I admit I've done my share of asking "why" over the course of my life. But God has taught me that a healthier question to ask is "What Now?" I have learned that it is not just what happens to you that counts, it is how you respond to what happens that makes all the difference in the world. And one way we develop strength of character is through various life situations and our responses to them.

I have been told that I have really been *lucky* to have survived a near death experience at age 12 and multiple surgeries over forty years with twenty-two joint replacements. However, my response is that I do not consider myself *lucky* but rather *I am blessed.* In my opinion, *luck* is another word for chance and is involved when drawing something out of a hat or flipping a coin.

When I consider my *Outlook* in life, I think more about what I call *Uplook*. Let me explain. Through our body (our earthly senses) and our soul (which includes our mind, emotions and will) we are continually perceiving and processing what we sense and experience. In addition to our body and soul, every human being also has a spirit that eventually yearns for more than this life can offer. I have discovered that a right relationship with God is the only true source of satisfying that yearning - and yes, each of us can have a personal relationship with the infinite God of the universe. But how can this be?

As Creator and Sustainer of all life, God the Father offers us His amazing grace and mercy through the sacrificial and atoning death of God the Son, Jesus Christ. When we acknowledge our own sinful nature, surrender our self-centered will, and place our faith in Jesus Christ, God forgives us and adopts us into His eternal family. We receive not only immeasurable spiritual blessings beyond death but are also given God's very present help in our earthly lives through the gift of His indwelling Spirit, God the Holy Spirit!

When I was young, I learned a simple definition of grace that captures its meaning: GRACE = **G**od's **R**iches **at** **C**hrist's **E**xpense. Even though God's grace is not something we can ever earn, it does involve an act of our will, a turning from our own self-centered ways and placing our faith in God's Way -Jesus. Jesus proclaims, "I am the way and the truth and the life. No one comes to the Father except through me." (*John 14:6, ESV*) Similar to the

GRACE acronym I also learned one for faith: FAITH = **F**orsaking **A**ll **I** **T**rust **H**im.

In more theological terms, the doctrine of salvation has been described by five Latin phrases that have come to be known as the Five Solas: *Sola Gratia, Sola Fide, Sola Christus, Sola Deo Gloria, and Sola Scriptura.* Translated it means salvation is "by grace alone, through faith alone, in Christ alone, for the glory of God alone, based on Scripture alone."

Finding my security, strength and hope from God helps me establish an overall balance in my life between what this earthly life holds and what is yet to come. Living with fear indicates I am trusting less in God and trusting more in my own limited understanding. When I recognize God's Presence is with me then I do not live in fear and anxiety of what tomorrow (or even today) holds. "For God has given us a spirit *not of fear,* but of power and love and self-control" (*2 Timothy 1:7, ESV*).

So, LOOKING UP *(Uplook)* to God as my Father in Heaven and trusting Him for my earthly and eternal life, shapes my LOOKING OUT (*Outlook*) at life. My *Uplook* impacts my *Outlook* in how I process life and allows me to look beyond the "why" of life's circumstances to instead focus more on "what now?"

I have been described by others as an extremely optimistic person. I like to think of myself as a realistic optimist. All in all, I am well-adjusted and am continuing to learn more and more about contentment in all circumstances, something about which the Apostle Paul challenges us when speaking in Philippians about one of his life lessons involving "learning to be content in every circumstance." (*Philippians 4:11, ESV*). I will share more about contentment in Chapter Six.

Despite the periods of adversity and the many challenges I have faced, I can truly profess that I have been and continue to be *blessed* – not *lucky*. Growing up, our family lived in a city where I could receive excellent medical care and I am especially grateful that God allowed me to live during a time of such great medical advancement. By the time I reached age twenty, the crippling effects of the disease were becoming a reality. Biomedical technology was at the point of introducing artificial hip replacements; however, I was initially not considered an appropriate candidate due to the fact that the projected life span of the replacement was around fifteen years. Thankfully, I had a progressive orthopedist who agreed to perform replacements in both of my hips. The surgeries were successful and over the next 45 years I underwent a total of 22 joint replacements - 18 total replacements and four partial replacements. In addition, I have had four replacement revisions and two re-replacements.

Several years ago, long after the death of my Mississippi orthopedist, I learned that he became well known in medical school textbooks for his accomplishments as a pioneer in joint replacement. My hip replacements, projected to have only a fifteen-year life span, are still intact with slight revision and are now 45 years old . . . and counting. Now that is what I consider a miraculous outcome that God accomplished through human skill and expertise!

With the care of excellent doctors, the love and understanding of those close to me and complete reliance on the Lord, I have led a remarkably active, productive, meaningful, and abundant life! I am also blessed to be married to my wonderful husband for almost four decades and together we are blessed with our only son whose precious wife we consider our "daughter-in-love."

However, this book is not meant to be all "sugar-n-spice and everything nice." I realize what it is like to be depressed and feel stuck in a miry pit. I also know what a joyous experience there is once you are lifted out of the pit. I have experienced the perspective you gain when viewing life from various mountaintops, as well as valleys and every step of the journey in between.

At the age of twelve, following emergency surgery and months of hospitalization, my arthritis recurred worse than ever, resulting in complications that, only with the Lord, I was able to handle. I felt that my life was being put on hold due to the need for institutionalized rehabilitation. However, in hindsight I recognized how God used that time and my experiences there to begin to teach me important life lessons about patience, endurance, and fortitude.

Then just five years later, at age seventeen, the unexpected death of my father brought more character-building opportunities and caused me to look more and more to God for my security and hope. I became more empathetic and grew in my understanding and compassion for others' suffering and life challenges. Additionally, I developed a keen awareness of the brevity of life. I learned that another key element in living a life of balance and contentment is appreciation of its short duration.

Leaving home for college just a year after losing my father also brought tremendous adjustments. I began to lean more on my Heavenly Father due to the loss of my earthly one. I also attribute a great portion of my growth and maturity during my college years to the nurture, guidance, love, and support that I received from my mother, even though she was deeply hurting as well. No other person had been through so much with me; no one else could understand me as she did; and nothing could ever surpass the tender love she so freely gave me.

Mother was a consistent and eloquent letter-writer. She was an executive secretary at a prominent law firm and took time each week to type me a letter before she left work for the day. At other times she handwrote letters, but I usually received at least one weekly letter or short note. These were a highlight to my week. I am including excerpts from some of the ones she wrote to me during my important college transition years. You can hear her heart, and from her comforting words you are able to detect her steadfast courage, her loving spirit, and her tender concern. The first letter is one that Mother sent me when I started college, and the other entries are excerpts from letters that I received from her throughout my college years.

> August 1975 – Freshman year
> My dearest Candy: You will already be at college when you read this. Yes, college, the next step in growing up, the step that your father and I have always dreamed of for both you and your brother. My prayer and concern is that we have equipped you for this step. You will live in a college atmosphere where you will be faced with so many temptations and it will be hard to be good. I hope you will always have a strong sense of what is truly right and truly wrong and have the courage and conviction to stand by it. So far, you have had this and I pray you will continue it in the future.

I know I have been carrying on about being lonely when you leave but I would be much sadder if you did not want to or were unable to go off to college, so even though I'll miss you greatly, I am happy in the thought that God has blessed you and you are able to go off to college. I have adjusted to many things in the past and will adjust to this too. So, don't feel sad or worry about me - just come home as often as you can. ha. As you know, I have joined several groups lately, and I plan to get myself a hobby of some kind to help fill my extra hours. You already know that I enjoy some time to myself anyway, so it will all fall into place.

I've tried real hard not to live your life for you or betray your trust in any way. I always wanted you to feel free to talk with me - not to the point of invading your privacy - just for you to feel the freedom of discussing anything with me. So, my point now is that no matter how tough a situation you might encounter or how disturbing it might be, just know that all you have to do is pick up your telephone and discuss it with me. Don't let me be the last to know what might be troubling you.

My daily prayer is that God will watch over you and take care of you and I know that you have many happy moments ahead of you. Of course, I love you more than my own life itself. Now, I'm getting "mushy," so I'll stop here. your loving Mother

<u>September 1975:</u> Candy, I hope you are settling down some by now and that you will not find your routine too tiring. I know you are facing a very "trying" time now, both with your adjusting to college, being away from home, and also over the changes that I anticipate making with selling the house and finding homes for the dogs. But just remember that this is life, and we find out what we

are made of when we have to face facts. You will undoubtedly be disappointed with many things and many people (maybe you are disappointed with some of my decisions), but I must do what I feel is best. You are making new friends and I must do the same thing. I cannot hold on to the past and the lonely memories. We must face the future with hope and faith that God will guide us correctly. I do pray that this coming week will be better for you and that all your adjustments will come a little easier. As you say, "Keep the Faith" and things are bound to get better! I love you, Mother.

March 1976 – The Following Spring, Freshman Year, Second Semester: Dear Candy, I was touched by some of the feelings you expressed in your last letter and whether you realize it or not, I do know something of what you are experiencing. You see, I lost my mother when I was not much older than you (and then had to adjust to another person taking her place, selling all my mother's household belongings, selling my home and all the things I loved so dearly).

So, you see, I do know something of your feelings. Of course, it is all part of growing up and facing the realities of life, and I am sorry that all this has hit you just when you are in the throes of college adjustment. You are making new friends, and even though you do not think so just yet, you are going to feel better as time goes by. I, too, would like to hold on to the past (much more than you realize, and I grieve for Dad much more than you and your brother realize), but I refuse to be morbid, and I refuse to go into a shell and ruin what life I have left. This would not be good for you, or for me.

Life constantly changes – sometimes for the best and sometimes not. I would like to think that our lives are changing for the best and I am doing all in my power to make a good life for us. I, too, always think about your health and it is one of my greatest concerns. I would give the whole world, if it were in my power, to have you feel good. I also know that the way you feel emotionally is sometimes caused by your health. It is extremely important that you take all your prescribed medication, get your rest, and eat right. These are key to your well-being.

I am glad that you expressed some of your inner feelings to me as this helps me to understand you (and vice versa). I hope you will always feel that you can communicate with me and that you will never feel that you have outgrown me. It breaks my heart when I see this happen to other people and I know they love their children the same as I do. You and your brother have always been the greatest thing that ever happened to your Daddy and me, and we have loved every minute of it. I pray for you each day - never would I miss it, as I know God does answer when we call upon Him. Love, Mother.

October 1976 – First Semester Sophomore Year:
I really did enjoy having you home this past weekend and will always look forward to your weekends home. I am extremely pleased over your apparent adjustment to everything under such very trying circumstances. I do know that if we ask God daily to help us that He will, and I'm counting on that. I hope this week will be a good one for you. Do take special care of yourself and be sure to eat right. I love you, Mother.

April 1977 – Second Semester Sophomore Year:
I will be remembering you in my prayers this week. I know you have been experiencing some traumatic times and I wish I could do something tangible to ease all the pain. Your visit with Dr. Purvis resulted in news that I know was hard for you to hear. You

have always valued your academics and that you view missing an entire semester to have surgery is a great interruption in your plans. However, if hip replacement surgery is what will help you walk without pain and keep you out of a wheelchair, then by all means your health comes first. I will just do what I can, and that is pray all will turn out for the best. Love, Mother.

March 1978 – Second Semester Junior Year, Following Hip Replacements in Fall 1977:
I hope this week has not proven to be too strenuous and that your tests were not so hard. I do really understand what a "trying" time you are having, still adjusting after your hip replacements. I think about you every day and every night. I know that you do have the "grit" to make it and that you are not a "quitter" so I'll just continue to pray that you will have the health and the stamina to hang in there. Do be careful. Remember that I love you, Mother.

February 1979 – Final Semester Senior Year:
Dear Candy (I love you): I don't see any reason why I should wait until the close of the letter to say "I love you" so I'll just start it off that way. Your beautiful valentine was waiting in my mailbox when I arrived home yesterday afternoon and the words are just beautiful. I know how much thought you put into selecting it and it meant that much more to me. I am so blessed to have two lovely, intelligent, and considerate children. I suppose Valentine's Day has brought out my sentimentality. Ha. I was sorry to hear that you feel so burdened down with your studies. I know it seems you have a lot on you but just try to do the best you can. Of course, the final phase of anything can be trying and now, of course, you are so looking forward to being out of school and getting on with your graduate schoolwork. Hope

this next week will be a good one for you, both physically and with your studies. Must run. I love you lots, Mother.

Thanks to Mother's prayers, understanding and consistent encouragement throughout my college years, and the difficult season of adjustment for the both of us in the loss of Daddy, I learned that change is not always bad and oftentimes necessary for growth. Like a plant that is pruned grows even heartier than before, so did these experiences, although painful at times, help me grow into a more positive, determined, and grateful person who recognized that God answers the prayers of a mother's heart. This would greatly impact my future role as a mother and also my personal commitment to prayer, which would become one of my life ministries!

Another influence Mother had on me was her positive and determined outlook on life. Like her, I was ambitious, always setting goals and striving to reach them. As for my personal goals, they were constantly being challenged, mainly due to my health limitations. "Hitch your wagon to a star," was one of my many mottoes.

When I first began college, I had the desire to study medicine and if I had been physically able, I would have pursued medical school. But things happen, and as lives adapt to circumstances, so goals may have to change.

During my sophomore year I decided to work toward applying to physical therapy school which seemed to be a natural choice. I had received therapy on numerous occasions and even volunteered in the physical therapy department as a hospital candy-striper (yes, I wore a red and white striped uniform and loved seeing people respond when I told them my name was Candy!)

I reasoned that the practice of physical therapy would give me contact with the medical field, as well as provide an opportunity for me to interact with and help people. Also, the educational curriculum would be less strenuous than medical school. BINGO! Once again, I had lassoed my career star and I had it within sight until my rope broke. My arthritic condition had worsened, and the crippling effects of the disease were rapidly becoming a reality. Deterioration of my hip joints reduced me to a cane with the prospect of a wheelchair on the horizon.

During the fall semester of my junior year, it became necessary to undergo two total hip replacements. I was only twenty years old. Having two major hip replacement surgeries during the same hospitalization, just ten days apart, meant a temporary halt in my education, and even more questions regarding my career path. While in rehabilitation following my hip replacements, in addition to physical therapy, I received occupational therapy.

New to me, I discovered that an occupational therapist works more with the functional and psychological rehabilitation of those who have trouble with life's normal daily activities due to injury, disease, or surgery. It involved adaptation and often innovation, two things I had been doing all my life.

So, what I had initially viewed as a major interruption in my life plan actually became the means for guiding me further in determining my career. I emerged from my recovery period with a stronger and more determined spirit than ever and continued to reach for those stars. My life's purpose was being revealed further. My desire of wanting to help people know and realize that their lives do not have to be hampered by illness, whether physical or mental, could be fulfilled! I looked for opportunities to learn more about the field of occupational therapy. My experiences during a period of volunteer work at a rehabilitation center inspired me to write the following:

> Life does make sense, sometimes . . . Today, due to my own previous suffering, I was able to understand the anguish of Chris, a spinal cord injury patient, as he struggled to put on his socks. I offered support as another patient angrily battled with buttoning his shirt. Less than nine months ago I could not reach my feet to tie my shoe. Fewer than three months ago I could not lift my arm to brush my hair. Because of my previous suffering, I can understand in a small way where Chris and Mike are coming from, and

possibly help them to understand where they are going. I'm thankful for my comings and goings and especially my "becomings." Life does make sense, sometimes. CC

With my career path established, I completed my undergraduate degree and moved to Texas for two and a half years of graduate study, completing my Master of Occupational Therapy degree in December 1982. I became employed as an occupational therapist and found great joy in giving people hope in the presence of despair and helping to instill desire and motivation where there were challenges and limitations. I was fulfilling a goal that gave me purpose and personal fulfillment, as I helped others realize that their lives don't have to be crushed by illness, destroyed by injury, or permanently halted by unwanted interruptions, whether physical, mental, emotional, circumstantial, relational, or even spiritual.

The role of my faith in Christ, a growing relationship with and dependence on God, as well as the various life circumstances I experienced, have all been factors in shaping my character, and have equipped me with the strength and perseverance I have needed to approach *each day anew*. And God's preservation of my life, despite numerous life-threatening complications along the way, became proof enough for me of the existence of a divine purpose for my life. Finding and fulfilling His will for me would become an ongoing process in itself - and not an easy or pain-free one.

In spite of many more surgeries that were to come and further life challenges and changes along the way, God continued to teach me the great benefits of not dwelling on the many "whys" of life but rather the forward moving, more hope-filled focus of "what now, Lord?" It is this kind of attitude that has helped me all along my journey to begin *each day anew.*

> ***Let us draw near to God***
> ***with a sincere heart***
> ***and with the full assurance***
> ***that faith brings . . .***
> ***Let us hold unswervingly***
> ***to the hope we profess,***
> ***for He Who promised is faithful.***
> ***Hebrews 10:22-23***
> ***(New International Version)***

# CHAPTER FIVE
## *Live, Love and Learn*

As we *live*, we will experience *love* in its various forms and if we are willing, we will *learn* many valuable life lessons. *Love is a Many-Splendored Thing* was a movie with a song in the soundtrack by the same name that rose to the top of the charts. It was the inspiration for the following poem about love that I wrote over 40 years ago. The poem was a wedding gift for one of my friends:

> Love is a many-splendored thing.
> A demonstration of caring, a lifetime of sharing.
> More giving than taking, and never forsaking.
> The kind of best friend who will be there to the end.
> Indeed, your love is a many-splendored thing!
> Love, Candy

Recently, I decided to look up the word *splendor* and found one of its meanings to be "magnificence" with synonyms including: grandness, grandeur, and brilliance. I have experienced a wide variety of love relationships over the years (with some NOT falling into the magnificent or grand category).

Our English word for love has so many different definitions and connotations. You can love your family and also love ice cream; you can love someone romantically or as a friend. Love can be fleeting or lifelong, it can be mutual or unreciprocated, it can be conditional or unconditional.

Some consider love a feeling, but I have learned that love goes much deeper than a feeling and involves a choice. (I plan to discuss feelings more in the next chapter.) Many writers and musicians have attempted to capture the meaning of love in word and song, as I did in my poem above, but the truth is that love is multi-faceted, and we can experience a variety of different kinds of love throughout our lifetime.

There are several Greek words for love that distinguish the various relationships and feelings we have for one another. Some resources list as many as nine uses and definitions. I recall learning about three basic types of love from Ancient Greek: *Phileo* (a general affection and loyalty toward friends), *Eros* (passionate, sensual desire, romantic love), and *Agape* (self-sacrificing, unconditional love).

C.S Lewis wrote about "the much beloved exploration of the nature of love" in his book, *The Four Loves,* and he describes a fourth love, *Storge.* It distinguishes familial love from *phileo*, the general affection toward a friend.

I've had friendships that have been close enough to be considered family. But there is still something mysteriously powerful about the connections we have with our biological family. *Storge* love is where I will begin, since my family is where I first lived, loved, and began to learn life lessons.

**Storge (Family Love)**

I was a "Daddy's girl," as the first chapter of this book, "*Little Princess*" indicates. I remember looking at early pictures of Mother and Daddy and thinking how handsome he was in his Navy uniform. Since his career was with the National Guard, he wore a crisply starched uniform every weekday and one weekend a month when he would "drill" with the local Guard unit. I always knew my daddy was an important and respected man, as many at his workplace and even some others outside work would often refer to him as simply "Colonel."

Daddy was affectionate and would let me sit in the recliner with him where I would smell the cherry pipe tobacco aroma from his clothing. When we would go to the beach where I was tentative about the waves knocking me down, he would let me ride piggy-back while he swam out past the breakers. Then he would float over the waves while I rode on his belly. He would also carry me on his shoulders to and from the creek at our family reunions, since I had city-folk tender feet and couldn't keep up with my excited, barefooted, country cousins running ahead of me through the wooded path that led to the creek.

On Saturdays, Daddy's attire was the one-piece jumpsuit that was so popular in the 60's & 70's. A special treat was when he would barbeque chicken on the specially made barbeque pit that he had made from half of an oil barrel drum. His famous secret barbeque sauce simmered all day and his barbeque process seemed to take hours, with him basting and turning the chicken so many times I would lose count. As we enjoyed his sauce-basted chicken, drenched with even more sauce as we ate it, we would kiddingly refer to it with the familiar motto from Kentucky Fried Chicken, "the Colonel's chicken is finger lickin' good!" I usually ended up with the sauce from ear to ear as well.

My time with Daddy was cut short when in 1974 he experienced a fatal heart attack and was gone in an instant. His death was especially traumatic because it occurred while I was away on a church mission trip in Ohio. The call to our youth minister came early on Sunday morning and I was whisked away to a small, local airfield where an Air National Guard transport plane landed.

My brother came down the flight of stairs to meet me with swollen red eyes and a hug that spoke more than words, confirming Daddy was gone. Our ride home was in the cockpit of that very loud propeller plane wearing headphones to drown out the noise, so no conversation was possible. Shock began to set in during that long flight home, and I remained that way for quite some time, as not only would I miss my daddy, but I would forever miss the way he loved me.

Even though I only had my daddy for seventeen years, God blessed me with my mother for 61 years, as she lived to be almost 93. Our relationship was more of a roller coaster one, as we were a lot alike and could easily push each other's buttons. Mother was fiercely independent, being a career woman by choice at a time when it was not the norm. But I never resented my mother for working.

Most of our really enjoyable memories were centered around shopping expeditions. Weekly grocery shopping trips involved teaching me about meal planning and list making. I especially enjoyed several wardrobe shopping expeditions we made each year – one for fall school clothes, another for Easter and spring outfits and then one for summer play clothes and swimsuits, which was my favorite. Even after I married, Mother would treat me to several "girls day out" shopping trips a year. Then one year the shopping trips shifted from adding to my own wardrobe to outfitting her long-awaited grandson. These were special times as well and much appreciated for our growing family's budget.

As I reflect on these things, I believe Mother's love language was giving gifts. But her gifts far exceeded material things. With Daddy gone, she was the one who spent countless hours by my hospital bed as my disease eventually required numerous surgeries and hospitalizations. As we both aged, and the roles reversed with my need to become her primary caretaker, it was sitting beside her hospital bed that I realized the many sacrifices she had made and the loving role model she had been for me.

My relationship with my brother, who was almost six years older than me, went through many stages. The story was told that he was so excited about having a baby sister and becoming a big brother that it took a great deal of convincing to get him to go back to kindergarten once I was born. He at least returned long enough to be in the Christmas play. One of my earliest memories with my big brother was how he would let me ride on his back, and I would squeal with delight when he became like a bucking bronco horse. Unfortunately, that game was halted when I fell off and hit my head hard enough to require stitches in my forehead.

As my brother entered his teenage years, I'm sure I became more like the pesky little sister. Daddy would allow my best friend and me to ride along in the front seat of the car as he chauffeured my brother and his girlfriend to school dances. I'm sure our giggles and kissing sounds made quite an impression. It was when my parents allowed him to begin babysitting me that revenge tickling sessions began. He would tickle me so hard and so long I would end up in tears, and my complaints to my parents that my big bad brother tickled me too hard didn't have the desired effect of my parents banning him from babysitting me again. As we became adults we grew apart, as he was always in a different life stage than me and we usually lived far apart. However, as Mother neared the end of her life, he really showed up for me. He is still the brother I adore, and there are more tender moments between us now.

*Storge* love, love that comes from family ties, is love that chooses you. It can be complicated at times, and sadly it can be dysfunctional or even abusive. Thankfully, I experienced the kind of familial love that withstood all kinds of trauma and trials and grew our bonds stronger, even when separated by time and distance.

## *Phileo* (Friendship Love)

I'm a people-lover, and every relationship, no matter what kind it happens to be, is just one more step along the path of life. Friendship relationships are so important. I've been blessed with more than my share over the years. Certain friends come into your life for a season and then you lose touch with them, however some relationships are forged deeper, and some are even lifelong. My lifelong friends are ones that I consider to be my "classic" friends, as I remember learning the definition of classic literature to be that which "withstands the test of time." Several of these from my childhood come to mind, my "sisters from another mother," who lost their mothers at relatively young ages and considered my mother as their second mother.

My backyard buddy was the closest to being a sister that I've ever had. She moved into our neighborhood during my early elementary years and only our backyards separated us from each other. Sleepovers, backyard plays, and holiday music recitals were some of our regular activities. Her family and mine shared in numerous joyous occasions, as well as deep sorrows over the years, and we still cherish times we get to spend together, even though distance now separates us.

Two of my high school girlfriends still hold a special place in my heart. One was a spunky, petite majorette in our high school band and her feature program included twirling fire batons. I was proudly her "fire baton lighter," and this role got me a place in the band (with an oversized band uniform which I proudly wore!) This fulfilled one of my childhood desires which had been to be a part of the band, since for years I had admired my older brother who had been band captain during his senior year in high school. Life took my "sister by choice" and me in different directions, but over the years we have remained one another's cheerleader when life events presented the need.

Another special friend from high school was the kind of friend that supported the concept that "opposites attract." She was much taller, I was short; she had long flowing hair and could wear the Farah Fawcett type haircut, mine was mostly short – more the Dorothy Hamill style. She was athletic, I was not; she was artistic, I was more the journalism type. But we had a great and loyal friendship – the kind that allowed for us to have other friends as well.

We attended college together and started out as college roommates. Even though we went separate ways in college. She pledged a sorority and I pursued classes with time consuming labs - our friendship remained. One memory that stands out is how we would take the school directory and look up boys' last names and try them out with our name to see if it would sound like a good married name. I decided that "Barr" would be a good married name to go with my name, Candy. I don't remember her favorite, but the funny thing is that she ended up marrying a guy with my maiden name. It was just like God to keep us connected with her getting my last name, even when I ended up not having it anymore. Thankfully, God rescued me from a lifetime of being "Candy Barr," for which I was especially grateful once I learned that she was a famous stripper from days gone by!

Throughout my college years, God also brought me a variety of friends, with a group of around 12 girls who ended up bonding and keeping in touch over the years. I fondly named us the "Dawgette Dozen" since we were Mississippi State Bull*Dawgs*. Many of my journal entries are from my college days:

> Thank God for friends. I was able to talk through some of my frustrations and it has helped me vent some emotions and bring them to the forefront so they can be dealt with. I am so grateful that my friends can help me come to grips with what I am feeling. That is what friendship is all about. Friends help you maintain your sanity by helping you acknowledge your feelings, whether they be right or wrong, and then by helping you deal with them.
>
> Friends come and go, which is all a part of the growing process. It is the friendship which manages to linger on, even when distance and circumstances result in separation. I never cease to be amazed how new friends continue to come into my life. But in new friendships, as well as old ones, times can get rough. I'm grateful God helps us work things out and grow from it.
>
> Another week of life, and it has really had its ups and downs. I'm really learning a lot about growing

relationships. My new friendships with two girls in the dorm grew a lot this week. We are experiencing growing pains, but that only signifies that growth is occurring. I pray for patience for each of us and for a willingness to try and understand each other and be of support. Above all, we really need that peace that surpasses all understanding, for those times when we can't understand...or won't.

Six weeks later:
Well, those growing pains six weeks ago really did signify growth. Those days of trials and tribulation were the germination period of seeds that are budding and beginning to bloom into beautiful friendships.

Various things inspired me to write during my early journaling years, but mostly I was inspired by people God brought into my life and special relationships that I experienced. You can see from the following poem how much my college friends meant to me and how big a part they played in my life. I wrote the following poem around the time of our college graduation in 1979:

### FRIENDS

The time has come, the work is done,
this chapter is at its end,
And our special times have meant so much more
cause we've shared them all as friends!

The ups, the downs, the ins, the outs,
the laughs and tears, the screams, and shouts.
All these things make life worthwhile,
and I can't help but crack a smile!

When I think of times we've spent in fun,
I'll cherish each and every one.
And when I think of every tear,
I'll remember those times and hold them dear.

But now this chapter must come to a close,
we're on to greater things.
There's jobs and schools and apartment life,
and even diamond rings!

We've finally grown up, the world is real,
the time to live is now.
The paths we take, the decisions we make,
are heavy ones, and how!

But let's all remember just one thing
as we go our separate ways,
It is memories and dreams and love and God
That will be with us ALWAYS!

CC 5-7-79

God continued to bring precious friends into my life during various seasons. My first big endeavor into apartment life I called "Westward Ho." In order to complete my graduate degree, I needed to move to Dallas, Texas. A relatively new friend was adventurous enough to accompany me to Texas and become my roommate. She was a classy lady but also practical, she liked trying new recipes and new restaurants. She was so compassionate and helpful to me personally. We both met our husbands while in Dallas, married just three months apart and ended up being each other's maid of honor. It was a special season in both of our lives. Even though we ended up living several states apart, we've made efforts to visit one another, and we are still just a phone call away.

Throughout various life stages of my adult years God brought incredibly special friends into my life. Fun couple times as YMNKs (Young Marrieds No Kids), then young moms with playdates for our kids. As our kids grew, we became homeroom moms, team moms and carpool moms. As soon as kindergarten began for my only son, I was drawn to a group of moms who gathered to pray for their children and their children's schools. It was these mighty prayer warriors who became some of my closest friends, and over twenty-five years later we still pray together in the Moms in Prayer ministry, lifting up to God our grown children and the challenges they are encountering in the chaotic and confusing world of today. In addition, we are encouragers to one another.

A poem I wrote many years ago speaks about how friends can really help you work through difficult times and emotions:

### WE DID IT, TOGETHER

I've finally stopped spinning around like a top
My taunt rubber band has decided to pop.
My music box mind has played out and wound down
And I've finally released my face from its frown.

For, a burden's been lifted
Things will work out for the best.
We prayed through it together,
Now I think I'll rest.


## GOD HAVE MERCY

God, have mercy on us when we manage
to screw our lives up so tight that we lose our cool
and blow sky high.

God, give us the strength and guidance
to work things out and go beyond the hurt
and rejection and misunderstanding.
God, give us the desire to have a softened heart
and a willing spirit, and
God, give us peace, whatever the outcome.

## *Eros* (My Romantic Experiences)

Choosing to love involves risk, especially where *Eros* or romantic love is concerned. It is easy to get all mushy and glassy-eyed and overlook the potential heartache that comes along with it. Many of my earlier journal writings contained poems which I wrote during a period when I was experiencing *unrequited* or *unreturned love*. I was in college and met a guy who was a great, personable, and fun person to be with. But he was oblivious to the depth of my feelings for him, and I allowed his behavior to greatly affect how I felt about myself. An excerpt from my journal demonstrated the challenges I experienced.

*Unrequited Eros Love:*

I wish I felt like I could cry. My emotions are so tensed up, I am numb. Anger, frustration, fear, hurt. I thought that I was angry, but actually I was hurt. It was fear of my feelings that caused my frustration. It was fear that everything was my fault and that I had brought the hurt upon myself, but then I realized I was wrong. All this time I thought it was my oversensitivity, when actually it was his insensitivity. I was calling his inconsideration, forgetfulness, and a carefree independent lifestyle, his need for room to breathe. No wonder I felt like I had brought it all on myself. I had done nothing but make excuses for him, but not anymore. Whether intentional or not, he has really hurt me. His inconsideration, insensitivity, and carefree existence have caused my heart to ache and my mind to face the reality that there is no excuse. What is so frustrating is the fact that in some weird way, no matter what my mind tells me, my heart still loves him, and that hurts. And because it hurts, it makes me angry. And that anger brings about fear, a fear that love doesn't conquer all – at least not *love that isn't returned*. I guess that is what hurts the most. When will I learn that love is not always a "many-splendored thing"? Sometimes it is downright rotten. At least the hurt won't last forever.

And at one point in this roller coaster relationship, I penned the following poem:

### DON'T BE AFRAID

Why can't you show me that you care?
Are you afraid of what you feel
   or don't you feel?

Are you hesitant as to what you might have to give up
or do you have no desire to give?
Perhaps I look for too much -
   a touch of compassion,
   a sign of concern,
   a simple call,
Just to let me know that you care.

Life would probably be much simpler
If I were to pretend
   that you don't care,
   that you don't feel,
   that you have no desire to give of yourself.
But I know those things aren't true.

Life is not meant to be simple,
   and neither are you.
Life is full of unanswered questions,
   and endless contradictions,
And so are you.

I'm not asking for more than you have to offer.
I'm just asking that you offer what you have.
That you not be afraid -
   to show me what you feel
   as long as it is real.

I care enough to know that you do care
   in your own way
   and in your own time.

It's just that one day
   your own way
     and your own time
       may be too late.

Don't be afraid to feel what is real.
Living is giving and caring is sharing.

So, share yourself with me.
   Show me that you care.
      *Don't be afraid.*

After I finished undergraduate school, I wisely left this relationship behind and set my sights on graduate school in Texas where new experiences and relationships awaited. The following poem expressed my state of mind following my relationship involving *Eros* love that wasn't mutual:

### I'M TIRED

I'm tired of table-scraps and leftovers
   and handouts when it's convenient.
I want to be treated like a queen
   and not like a puppy begging
      for a pat on the head.
I want to feel loved and important
   and wonder why someone cares about me,
      not why he doesn't.
Is that too much to ask?

## <u>Unequally Yoked Eros Love</u>

During my years at graduate school, I returned home intermittently for surgeries on my shoulders and elbows. One summer toward the end of one of my recovery periods, a friend and I enjoyed a getaway to the beach. To my great surprise I met a guy working there at our resort who took a liking to me, thus a summer romance ensued and even continued once I returned home. In all of his romantic pursuits he even hitchhiked 150 miles from the beach to my home to surprise me with a proposal and a promise ring! I was so caught up in the fairy tale experience of someone finally caring enough to pursue me that I was swept off my feet.

However, once I returned to Texas where I was surrounded by my highly educated peers and a strong Christian fellowship, God began to reveal reality and truth. I realized that my new relationship was one described by the Apostle Paul as one where we were *"unequally yoked" (2 Corinthians 6:14, ESV)*. When my Prince Charming visited me in my normal surroundings, reality hit him too. Before long, our engagement was broken and so were both our hearts.

When a relationship ends and two people part, it's hard to see the good apart from the pain. Yes, I had experienced a relationship where I was finally cared for and romanced, however *unequally yoked* love can also bring heartache. I'm grateful God revealed the truth before we made the mistake of marrying. God also revealed to me that all relationship experiences can bring growth and are a part of learning to begin *each day anew*. Time does help heal broken relationships. After a time of healing, I was able to write the following poem about this special fellow:

## THINKING OF YOU

When I think of happiness and laughter
   and a sunshiny day filled with smiles,
     I'll think of you.
When I think of caring and sharing
   the ups and the downs and all arounds,
     I'll think of you.

It's your unique style
   that makes knowing you worthwhile,
You make life an adventurous game.
And for those lives you touch
   with your lively nonsuch,
They are really quite never the same!

So . . .
When I think of life's blessings,
   That are meant to be just for a time,
When I think of laughter
   and sharing and caring,
     I'll always think of you!

I refocused my energies toward completing my graduate studies, and continued to journal which really helped me process various things that God was teaching me about *Eros* love relationships:

> God, you have taught me about love through allowing me to experience relationships with two fellows, one who didn't return my love and another who pursued me but wasn't the right one for me. These relationships came to an end, but they have all been a part of my learning more about love. One thing I have learned is that you can love someone without being "in love." I truly still love these guys

even though my expectations for our relationships were not fulfilled. Another revelation is the fact that you don't "fall in love or out of love," rather it is a growing process which can take time. Teach me how to be content with Your timing, Lord!

It an extremely important fact in life that you must be happy and content and love yourself before any healthy relationship can develop with others. Just look around and those who are unhappy with their relationships with others and are bitter at the world are probably unhappy with themselves.

I know now, with all my heart, that I cannot and must not continue expecting others to be "that certain someone" just meant for me. I must make sure my own life is free and independent and following the guidance and direction of the Lord, and then all else will fall into place, even my relationships. I am learning that being an individual is merely the fulfillment and expression of God's creation and we are made first and foremost in His image. We're not to build our lives around another person, only our love for God. Only when we realize *whose* we are can we begin to really discern *who* we are, and only then can we begin to build healthy relationships with others.

I came across the following saying, and it really speaks to my desire for a lasting love relationship: "If you want something very, very bad, let it go free. If it comes back to you, it is yours forever. If it doesn't, it was never meant to be yours at all." I must let this yearning for a life mate go free and if I am meant to have such a relationship it will happen and come to me in God's timing.

A brief but poignant journal entry was entitled:

> SO THEY SAY
> Love isn't easy
> but it's worth it
> so they say . . . we'll see.

## *Unexpected True Love*

At a time and in a way that was *unexpected,* God brought the man into my life who would become my husband. I had always looked forward to developing a love-filled and long-lasting relationship where caring means sharing and living means giving. The kind of love that goes beyond sensual desire and incorporates friendship and unconditional love. And God richly blessed me by giving me a marriage where true love exists and grows daily. The following poem was written to capture the simple pleasure of true love and its many aspects.

### SIMPLY BECAUSE . .

When I receive a letter or a card
    and it's from you -
I read what it says,
    and warmth fills my heart,
    and my face begins to smile,
Simply because . . .I like it when you say, "I love you."

When the telephone rings
    and it's you -
I hear your voice,
    and sunshine fills my day,
    and my spirit is lifted,
Simply because . . . I like when you say, "I love you."

When we're together, arm in arm, alone and quiet,
I feel your gentle touch,
    and peace and joy fill my soul,
    and my life is made complete,
Simply because... I like it when you say, "I love you."

So, whether we're together or apart,
    You will always be in my heart,
Simply because... I love you, too!
      All my love, Candy

## *Storge* (Family Love) The Circle of Life

I married in my late twenties, and due to my rheumatoid arthritis and the medications I took, I was uncertain if I would be able to have children. After five years of marriage, a career move from Texas to Alabama, and having both of my knees replaced, it was time to seriously consider the parenthood decision. I had many fears and feelings of inadequacy about the issue – regarding conception, my health during pregnancy, health of the baby, limitations regarding my ability to physically handle an infant and small child, the extra stress and demands it would require of my husband – just to name more than a few!

It came down to whether we trusted God enough and genuinely believed that if He allowed us to conceive then He would provide us with whatever we needed to parent, not only through the early years but throughout the entire parenting process.

Once we consulted with my physicians and took the necessary steps to eliminate medications that could be harmful to the baby, God allowed us to conceive, and my pregnancy went better than we could have imagined. I only gained 13 pounds and was all baby, which made it less stressful on my joints. Our healthy baby boy arrived in time for us to bring him home on Christmas Eve, which gave new meaning to the emotions surrounding the earthly arrival of the Christ Child.

There were indeed extra parenting challenges for us with my physical limitations, but with some adaptations, a great support system and a very invested and amazing husband, God was faithful to reveal His provisions every step of the way. And we have come to realize how parenting throughout all seasons of our children's lives brings challenges, but the blessings far outweigh the difficulties!

### *Agape* (Unconditional Love)

Becoming a parent and all it involves, in addition to the other types of love relationships that I've described so far, can teach us many things. Human relationships can meet certain needs we have for love, but what our souls most yearn for is *Agape* love. *Agape* is an unconditional love, the source of it being God and the unconditional, undeserved love He has for us.

Christianity is not just a religion or set of beliefs about God, rather it centers on the love God has for us and the relationship we can have with Him. Because God first loved us and gave His Son for us while we were still sinners, we can enter a relationship with God and live as His beloved children. The growing Christian begins to reflect God's *agape* love towards others. We love because God first loved us (*1 John 4:19, ESV*). *Agape* love is an intentional choice and expressed not only to those who agree with us, but to those with whom we have differences, disagreements or even dislike. This kind of love can weather the storms of conflict and even enable us to pray for our enemies.

Caring is important but sharing goes even farther in demonstrating *Agape* love. A caring person who is open to sharing is willing to take off his mask and let others see who he really is. This takes courage and requires trust, but the person who practices openness and trust will find that others will be more open and trusting as well. I consider the first cousin to openness to be honesty. The honest person who cares about others gets in touch with what he thinks and how he truly feels, then shares his feelings at appropriate times and in appropriate ways.

I am convinced that open, honest communication is one aspect of *Agape* love and provides a strong foundation for healthy relationships. This begins in our relationship with God, through open, honest prayer, and then it can impact every other relationship we have – whether the relationships are with our family (*storge*), our friends (*phileo*) or in our romantic relationships *(eros)*. Especially when our *Eros* relationships are grounded in *Agape* love, then authentic caring and sharing, along with open and honest communication, will guide our hearts according to what God intends.

In reflecting on some of these relationships that I've experienced throughout the years, I have learned how important relationships are and how they must become a priority in our lives. Our relationship with our Creator and Sustainer of life is foundational and impacts how we respond in every other relationship and situation we encounter.

When Christ came to earth, He was the embodiment of *Agape* love and called His followers to a higher standard of love than merely loving others as we love ourselves. In the gospel of John, Jesus is recorded as saying, "A new commandment I give to you, that you love one another; *just as I have loved you, you are also to love one another.* By this all people will know that you are my disciples if you have love for one another" *(John 13:34-35, ESV)*. The role of forgiveness is also one of the things we need to establish healthy relationships – both with God and with others.

It is only through God's unconditional, unfailing, and eternal love for me that I can risk loving others and investing in the relationships He brings into my life. It is also the reason that I have courage to begin *each day anew*! So live, love and learn!

***So now faith, hope and love abide, these three.***
***But the greatest of these is love.***
***1 Corinthians 13:13***
***(English Standard Version)***

# CHAPTER SIX
## *How Do You Feel?*

"How are you feeling today?" I've encountered this question countless times in my life, especially since I've had a chronic disease. Most people do not really expect details or mean to delve into my innermost feelings when they ask this question. Even if they are genuinely interested, most of us interpret the question to relate to our physical state and many of us are so out of touch with our emotions that we would have difficulty genuinely answering the question. So, usually the easy, efficient, and polite answer is "Fine" or "Okay" or possibly even "So-So." How do we actually determine how we feel? Let's explore this.

God created us with a physical body which includes senses that enable us to interpret and relate to our environment. What we see, hear, smell, taste and touch are integral parts of our human development and learning. Even physical pain is important as a protective mechanism and can be a red flag when something about our bodies needs attention.

We are also created with a soul which encompasses our will, our mind, and our emotions, which many call feelings.

Thought, emotion and decision-making abilities are all a vital part of how we engage and respond to the people and situations in our lives. Many of my initial journal entries were expressions from my soul and the topics were mostly about relationships and circumstances that I was experiencing. One thing writing has done for me is to give me an outlet to get my thoughts and feelings down on paper while they are fresh. It gives me practice in learning how to identify what I'm thinking and feeling and then process them further in a way that helps me maintain a healthy balance.

Over the years I have experienced times when my emotions did get out of balance, and it was more than just "that womanly time of the month." I call it feeling "out of sorts." In times like these, emotions can run wild and can become all consuming. They can even become the driving force in our reactions and decisions. When this occurs, we are more likely to experience an unhealthy balance in our soul which can drastically impact the health of our physical bodies.

Emotions, when identified and processed in a healthy way, can be the source of many valuable lessons. However, we must be willing to admit what we are feeling, work to process our emotions and be willing to learn from them. I've experienced a wide variety of emotions over the years and some of my early journal examples demonstrate a few:

On a blue day...

> I feel like crying my insides out. My emotions are just about shot. The days just past have been very trying. Lord, are you telling me something? Why the recent disappointment on top of disappointment? Must I start over again? Must I wipe the slate clean and give it another try?

But the sun does shine again...

> I'm really glad that I'm getting in touch with my feelings these days. God is giving me the strength to discern between my feelings of dependence and independence. My perspective is getting clearer and clearer every day. Until I heard myself giving others advice that I should take myself, did I really begin to listen. I was still clinging to another someone more than I was to God and as much as I told myself I was my own person, independent and free of anyone else, it still was not true. Who was I fooling? No one, not even myself, and especially not God. Perhaps God is the only one I should be clinging to.

And lessons are learned...

> I cannot change my heart, only God can do that. But I can become more aware of my emotions, work on my attitude, and control my actions, especially my reactions. Words have come from my mouth many times over, but until an experience brings those words into plain view and clear focus, the heart does not really respond. Even though I have told myself certain things over and over, I never really believed them, or let myself believe them with all my heart... until my heart became directly involved. Grateful that the God of all comfort who comforts us in all our afflictions hears my heart and heals all hurts!

This leads me to discuss the third aspect of how we are created. In addition to having a body and a soul, we have a spirit. Our spirit is perhaps the most mysterious part of our entire being. It is the part of us that relates beyond the natural realm to the supernatural realm. Our Creator made us with a body from the dust of the earth, which He created in His image; and a soul within our bodies that thinks, feels, and has freedom of choice. He also breathed His breath into our bodies, placing a sense of eternity in our souls *(Ecclesiastes 3:11, ESV).* This is our spirit.

Within our spirit is an innate sense that there is more to our lives than what we experience through our physical senses or emotions and exceeds what we can reason with our minds. Our spirit is the part of us designed to relate beyond our senses and intellect through what is considered to be our faith. An important question of our lives becomes who or what do we place our faith in beyond ourselves and our earthly lives?

I have previously referenced The One and Only True and Living God, who is not only Creator God but is also my Heavenly Father who knit me together in my mother's womb *(Psalm 139:13, ESV).* I experienced physical birth when it came time for me to be delivered into my earthly family. My early years were filled with amazing growth and development - body, and soul. Then at age 10, I experienced a "second birth" as my spirit was awakened, and I placed my faith in Christ.

It was then that I began a spiritual and personal relationship with Christ, who is also known as the Son of God as well as the second person of the Triune God (The Trinity). History records how Christ became a human, lived on earth, willingly gave His life to fulfill the penalty for all mankind's sin, and redeemed us from physical death and eternal destruction, restoring our broken relationship with the Creator God, our Heavenly Father.

So, by God's grace and through faith in Christ, I received the gift of the Holy Spirit, who is the third person of the Trinity. He supernaturally resides in my spirit as a guarantee of the hope that exists far beyond what my body and soul can experience in this life. Through the help of the Holy Spirit, I can learn about such things as joy in the midst of suffering, peace that passes all understanding and even true contentment while I live on earth. And more importantly, my life does not end with physical death but rather my soul and spirit will be eternally present with God forever!

Through my body, soul, and spirit I have learned that my feelings and the circumstances in my life, as well as my faith, are all complementary in learning how to acknowledge and process what *happens* in my life and how to *handle what happens.* Many consider *happiness* to be their ultimate goal in life. Even in the Declaration of Independence, our forefathers established the importance of *the pursuit of happiness.*

Happiness is affected by many factors such as health, relationships, the environment, one's income, and especially personal expectations and a sense of control. I have found *happiness* to be fickle and elusive because it largely depends on what *happens.* I have discovered that aiming for a healthy balance in my life is a much better goal than the pursuit of happiness. This healthy balance I'm referring to is not merely *a feeling of happiness* but rather *a state of being called contentment.*

Contentment has been defined as "a state of satisfaction and acceptance of circumstance, in spite of the pain or discomfort involved." In William Barclay's The Secret of Contentment, he states that contentment must be learned and comes from knowing God and delighting in His sovereign goodness and fatherly care. The apostle Paul declared through his various circumstances, even suffering, that he had learned to be content in whatever situation he encountered *(Philippians 4:11, ESV).*

Through many decades of my life, there have been various lessons along the way, teaching me about contentment. In looking back over my journal entries, as well as recalling seasons of my life where I learned the most valuable lessons, I discovered that I learned the most through painful and difficult circumstances – usually associated with various kinds of loss. I've grouped these types of loss into three categories: Loss due to *disease* and its impact, loss through *death* of a loved one, and loss experienced with *depression* or mental health challenges.

**Loss Due to Disease**

As I begin writing about this topic, I am actually 3 months out from a fall that broke my thigh bone near my hip replacement that is 44 years old. It required extensive reconstructive surgery in an effort to preserve the hip implant and avoid having to remove it and attempt another replacement. With bone grafts used to supplement the bone that had been splintered, it has been necessary to remain off the leg with no weight bearing this entire time in order for the bone to begin fusing together. This has meant spending most of the time in my recliner, with someone having to physically transfer me to the wheelchair, the bed and yes, even the bedside commode.

Post-op recovery isn't something that is new to me, however with previous joint surgeries, rehabilitation began much sooner and by three months I have usually progressed to the point where I am functioning mostly independently, with just a few limitations, if any. Functional ability is something most of us take for granted and when something in our lives disrupts our daily function it can result in varying degrees of loss. The key words in reference to this kind of loss are *dependence* and *limitation*.

I am one who likes to be in control. Perhaps you are too. I've realized that some of my tendency to want to control comes from having to face times in my life where I experienced loss of control. Because of the diagnosis of juvenile rheumatoid arthritis when I was a young child, I encountered a variety of frustrations associated with *dependence, limitation, and loss of control*. Disease flares, as well as the need for surgical intervention, brought periods where certain aspects of my life would become beyond my control.

The need for extra rest, as well as physical limitations when my joints would become swollen and painful, kept me from participating in activities my friends were doing, such as pep squad, sports teams, and marching band. Recurring needs for surgeries brought interruptions to my personal plans more times than I can count. When a hip, knee or foot is involved, the ability to move freely when and where you want to go, is compromised. When there is a shoulder, elbow, or hand out of commission, very quickly function and independence becomes limited. Simple but important activities such as eating, showering, brushing your teeth or your hair, and pulling your pants up and down, are just a few of the things that can result in the need for help. This really challenges your sense of independence.

Other diseases can bring a different set of challenges, such as diabetes or heart disease which can require a variety of major lifestyle changes. Life-threatening diagnoses such as cancer, multiple sclerosis and ALS involve not only major changes, but also evoke a set of fears and unknowns that can become mentally and emotionally paralyzing. It becomes understandable how one's focus can easily and quickly shift from temporary limitation and dependency to loss, anger, resentment, and depression.

I wrote the following poem during the period in college prior to accepting that I needed to undergo hip replacement surgery. I was really hurting, physically, mentally, emotionally, and spiritually.

## GOD, IT HURTS

God, I am really hurting . . .
    inside and outside,
    emotionally and physically,
    mentally and spiritually.
I guess that covers just about every aspect of my life.

Why must I hurt so badly?
And for what seems such a long period of time?
Is this what you mean by "long-suffering"?

GOD, I am really weary . . .
    in body,
    in soul,
    and in spirit.
I keep thinking that the burden
    is about to become unbearable,
But for some reason it doesn't, it just hurts.

When will the burden be lifted?
When will the hurt go away?
When will it begin to make sense?

GOD, I really want Your will in my life . . .
    with all my heart,
    with all my mind,
    and with all my strength.

I trust that You are directing my path.
I believe that You are working
all things together for good.
I do love You and want to seek
Your purpose for my life.

Help me to trust You more,
    to believe Your promises more,
    to love You more, in spite of the hurt.

GOD, Heal my hurt.
    Sustain me with Your peace,
    Fill me with Your joy,
Guide and direct me in Your infinite wisdom and love,
And remind me always . . .
    that YOU HURT TOO.

## Loss Associated with Death

Death often gives us a keener perspective on life. As quoted by Tagore in *Stray Birds*, "Death belongs to life as birth does. The walk is in the raising of the foot as in the laying of it down." The following poem which I wrote shortly after my father's death, expressed my increased awareness and appreciation of life, acknowledging the importance of embracing both the highs and lows. A study of sonnets in English gave me the challenge of writing one of my own.

### LIFE'S SONNET

Life is filled with many joys and heartaches
Ask anyone you know; they'll tell you so.
There are times of peace when rowing on calm lakes,
There are times to cheer you up when you feel low.

Life deals harsh blows when least expected to,
But also gives you strength to ease the pain.
Life's like a cloud that hides the sky so blue,
But also like the sun that clears the rain.

O Life, how very precious is each breath
Granted by our Creator up above.
Conceived and birthed and lived until your death,
Experienced, all the more, when filled with love!

Life, so wonderful, so short, so lovely.
Make a person grateful that he has thee.

We often describe the death of someone close to us as the *loss* of a loved one. Indeed, there is a great sense of loss when we no longer have that person in our lives, especially in relationships where we were close. Even divorce or a permanent break-up can result in the death of a special relationship that brings a great sense of loss. Grief is a normal and very important process that can include a number of stages as described by psychologists. These may include shock and denial, anger and bargaining, a period of depression, and hopefully eventual acceptance and renewed hope. These stages of grief can also apply to losses other than just death.

As described previously in my battle with chronic disease, responses such as anger, resentment, and depression are common. Often when life-changing diagnoses are received, denial may even be an initial response. It is when acceptance of reality occurs that the hard work of moving through and beyond the loss can result in a healthy grief process. Everyone is unique and therefore each person may respond differently in how loss is handled.

## **Loss Experienced with Depression:**

A different kind of loss that I've personally experienced is when I found myself in the dark and miry pit of depression. The kind of depression where you lose a sense of yourself, and you can no longer function as you normally do. Loss of sleep, loss of appetite, loss of concentration, loss of confidence, loss of the ability to plan or see a positive future, are all part of the depression I have lived *through*. And the important word here is *through*. Just as grief is a process, so is the journey *through* depression.

When your brain chemistry gets out of balance, your brain function can actually "depress" and so can your other body systems. Understanding this fact de-stigmatizes the need to seek professional help. A proper diagnosis and medication, when indicated, can help re-establish a healthy balance of brain function. Other supportive therapies can also help provide coping mechanisms to restore functional abilities.

The sense of being "stuck" with no hope of getting better can be a paralyzing aspect of depression. The most helpful coping skill I learned, which still serves me well, is "Just do the next thing." It may be as simple as pulling back the covers to get out of bed or focusing on getting a shower or walking into the kitchen to get something simple to eat. Soon "the next thing" becomes a string of next things that free you from the inertia that can accompany depression.

Depression can also decrease your appetite for eating as well as life in general. Ways I found helpful to combat these symptoms were to go ahead and eat foods or do things I knew I once enjoyed, even though I didn't feel like it. As I did, the activity helped stimulate positive brain chemicals which helped me return to being able to eat and be active again.

As with loss due to the impact of a life-changing disease or grief over the loss of a loved one, encouraging someone battling depression does not come in the form of "Oh, I wish you didn't feel so bad," or "It could be much worse," or "You just need to get on with your life." Rather, it is best to look for practical ways to lend a helping hand. Simple things can help such as showing up to wash dishes, help with laundry, or go for a walk or drive. Even just calling to let them know you're thinking about them and offer to run errands or accompany them to an appointment can be helpful. Just listening to the voice of a friend on my answering machine, when I didn't feel up to answering the phone, brought me encouragement because I knew they were there for me.

It may seem that experiences with disease, death, and depression are all loss and no gain. But I disagree. Think about the caterpillar, that after a certain period of enjoying life, satisfying its appetite in eating all it wanted, there comes a time where it enters a dark and lonely phase of life inside a cocoon. Life as the caterpillar has known it is over and it may seem that no hope of any future exists. But a miraculous transformation is occurring, even during this dark and seemingly endless stage of life. At the proper time, a break in the darkness finally comes, and a struggle ensues to break free of the cocoon. The cocoon was only a stage of life, not the end of life. In fact, the transformation that has taken place and the struggle to emerge from the restricting darkness actually brings forth new beauty and ability!

The strength of the butterfly's new wings comes only from its struggle to enter the light. Now the butterfly is free to fly and experience things it never could as a caterpillar. In essence, life did not end during the dark phase of the butterfly's life, nor was the most fulfilling part of its life in being a caterpillar. We must ask ourselves, is life's struggle something to avoid or is the strength that comes from the struggle worth it?

A quote from *Hinds Feet on High Places* by Hannah Hurnard has been in my journal for years:

> As Christians, we know, in theory at least, that in the life of a child of God there are no second causes, that even the most unjust and cruel things, as well as all seemingly pointless and undeserved sufferings, have been permitted by God as a glorious opportunity for us to react to them in such a way that our Lord and Savior is able to produce in us, little by little, his own lovely character.

God is the God of all comfort and helps us through every situation in our lives. One of the great comforts is that nothing in our lives is wasted. One of God's many promises to those who love Him and are called according to His purpose, is that He will work all things together for good *(Romans 8:28, ESV)*. However, our perception of good can often be extremely different from God's. He tells us, "For my thoughts are not your thoughts, neither are my ways your ways, declares the Lord. For as the heavens are higher than the earth, so are my ways higher than your ways and my thoughts than your thoughts" *(Isaiah 55:8-9, ESV)*.

I continue to be reminded that my life is a process and not to be measured by the world's values of success and failure; rather it is grounded in the fact that I have an all-powerful, all-knowing, and trustworthy Heavenly Father. He created me, loves me and through His Son, Jesus, has given me the gift of eternal life. Additionally, I have been given His Holy Spirit who is present with me and is at work in me and through me for my good and God's glory! When I remember these truths, I gain courage to approach once again *each day anew*.

**For the LORD is good;**
***His steadfast love endures forever,***
***and His faithfulness to all generations.***
**Psalm 100:5**
***(English Standard Version)***

# CHAPTER SEVEN

## *Look Within:*
## *Time to Rest and Reflect*

In the fast-paced world of today, time seems to be something we never have enough of. We are always in a hurry running here and running there, slaves to the clock and always using the excuse, "I don't have the time." We are an activity-oriented culture but let us remember that we are first and foremost human <u>beings</u> not human <u>doings</u>. As we determine how to use our time each day, it is important to intentionally make time to be still, to rest, and to reflect.

Rest is important to renew our bodies, our souls, and our spirits. What is restful for one person may be different from what someone else finds to be restful. Rest can be as simple as pushing your own personal pause button for a few minutes to practice deep breathing and relaxation imagery. Time spent out in nature, taking a walk, watching the birds, or a simple change in scenery, can also be restful. For some reading a good book or listening to music helps to relax and rest. And don't forget about the value of a good afternoon nap, one which I personally hated as a kid but look forward to now as an adult. These are examples of rest that primarily renew our physical bodies.

Rest for our soul and spirit usually requires carving out a more intentional time to focus our minds away from our "to do list" and to quiet ourselves long enough to reflect and *"Look Within."* My "quiet time" often includes communicating my thoughts and even my prayers, in writing. My more meaningful journal writings occurred only when I took the time to be still, to pause from my regular activity and to allow myself to reflect upon life. The following represent some of these entries:

> This first day of the new year has been a very settled and contemplative one. I started the year with family and friends. I wonder with whom I will end it? Exciting times ahead, lots of living to do, but for now I must rest while I can.

> It's been a quiet day. It is good to be alone sometimes and to take time to think about life, meditate on God's Word, and converse with Him through prayer, listening more than talking. That's when you get to know yourself better - and God!

> I must learn to appreciate time to myself. A lot of my time this past weekend was spent alone -- time I really needed for myself. I'm trying to really examine myself and my priorities and make commitments where I need to. Getting to know God better really helps. Lord willing, and my spirit willing, I will be able to commit my time and effort where it can be of best use, both to God and to me.

I am fervently searching and asking God to reveal Himself to me through whatever means He should choose and therein I will commit myself and my efforts. If it is in healing me, in giving me the strength to endure, in giving me peace in spite of my inability to understand, or whatever, I'm ready to listen. I just have to be still and take time to block out the noise in my life so I can hear when His Spirit speaks.

My days are long. I'm so weary that I'm sick to my stomach. The anxiety of what lies ahead in the next few weeks is about to get too good of a hold on me. I must rest and let God take this burden off my shoulders.

Even though my body is weak, and my mind is tired, I know God will strengthen me daily. I realize more and more the importance of allowing Christ to be Lord of my life and not just my Savior. I have some heavy things coming up next week so I'm really lifting these next few days and weeks up to the Lord. I'm also working on contentment without romance, which is becoming one of my greatest weaknesses. I pray for a calming spirit in that realm of my life. Oh, for a peace beyond all understanding to sustain me. Praise God for the strength to endure!

Many times, God has a firm hand in our life decisions and situations, and at other times He wants us to decide things on our own. God can even work in our lives in new ways by saying NO and NOT YET. I want my timing to be God's timing. I am confident that God will guide me, and just that fact alone, without knowing anything else, can bring me comfort and peace.

As I review these journal writings from over forty years ago, some things make me smile, especially when life done God's way is made to sound so simple, like "I want **my** timing to be God's timing." As a young adult, I still had to learn that life is not all about me and **my** timing, hoping that God's timing agreed with mine. More often than not I found that God's timing did not at all line up with mine. On a number of occasions when life events such as a joint replacement surgery became a necessity, I considered the forced downtime during the recovery periods to be a major interruption in my own life plans. Even as I write this, I have not been able to walk for nine months due to a fall and subsequent reconstruction surgery and I am facing a follow-up surgery as well, so more waiting to hopefully walk again. An abridged version of a favorite poem of mine by Russell Kelfer is about the value of waiting.

### WAIT

I pled and I wept
for a clue to my fate,
and the Master so gently said,
"Child, you must wait."

"Wait, You say, wait?"
was my indignant reply.
"Lord, I need answers,
I need to know why?"

## EACH DAY ANEW

"My future and all
to which I can relate,
hangs in the balance,
and You tell me to WAIT?"

Then quietly, softly,
I learned of my fate,
as my Master replied once again,
"You must wait."

So, I slumped in my chair,
defeated and taut
and grumbled to God
"So, I'm waiting . . . for what?"

He seemed then to kneel,
and His eyes wept with mine,
and He tenderly said,
"I could give you a sign."

"All you seek I could give you
and pleased you would be.
You would have what you want
but you wouldn't know Me."

"You'd not learn to see
through the clouds of despair.
You'd not learn to trust
just by knowing I'm there."

"You'd not know the joy
of resting in Me
When darkness and silence
were all you could see."

"You'd not know My comfort
late into the night.
The faith that I give
when you walk without sight."

"You never would know,
should your pain quickly flee,
what it means that
My grace is sufficient for Thee."

"Yes, your hopes and prayers
overnight would come true.
but, Oh, the loss if I lost
what I'm doing in you!"

"So, be silent, My Child,
and in time you will see
that the greatest of gifts
is to get to know Me."

"And though often My answers
may seem terribly late,
My most precious answer of all is to
BE STILL AND WAIT."

Periods when our lives seem interrupted, sidetracked with a detour, or even at a standstill, are never time that is wasted. In fact, when being still is imposed rather than voluntary, I may finally get the rest that I didn't realize I needed. It could be divine re-direction and time to re-examine my intended goals or purpose, or it may even be time for an adjustment in my attitude or expectations.

Some of my greatest frustration comes from unmet expectations. Our personal expectations, other's expectations, circumstances, and the demands of daily living can result in moments, days and even months when life may seem out of control. And for the most part, life IS beyond our control. An exception includes our personal responsibility and self-control and even then, there are times we may lose that.

The effort we make to keep all the parts of our lives together and running smoothly can become all-consuming, and the result we achieve is not really what brings true satisfaction. God promises that we can live through the not so perfect aspects of our lives, and even the most difficult times and events, and still be centered, steady, peaceful, and content. But it is a learning process. Even the Apostle Paul, a great hero of the Christian faith, tells us, "I have learned in whatever situation I am to be content." (Philippians 4:11b, ESV).

Corrie Ten Boom is one of my faith heroes. Things happened in her life that were certainly unexpected and beyond her control, even atrocious. Corrie's family helped the Jews during the reign of Hitler, and subsequently members of her family were sent to and died in concentration camps. Corrie survived, and her story has been told in book and film, entitled *The Hiding Place*. Corrie spent the remainder of her life traveling the world and giving her testimony regarding forgiveness and God's amazing grace. One of her written reflections is extra special to me and one I recall frequently when life becomes challenging:

## LIFE IS BUT A WEAVING
## (THE TAPESTRY POEM)

My life is but a weaving
Between my God and me.
I cannot choose the colors,
He weaveth steadily.

Oft' times He weaveth sorrow,
And I in foolish pride,
Forget He sees the upper
And I the underside.

Not 'til the loom is silent
And the shuttles cease to fly,
Will God unroll the canvas
And reveal the reason why.

The dark threads are as needful
In the weaver's skillful hand,
As the threads of gold and silver
In the pattern He has planned

He knows, He loves, He cares.
Nothing this truth can dim.
He gives the very best to those
Who leave the choice to Him.

With spending most of the past year in forced downtime, I've had more than my share of time for rest. Therefore, I've composed an acronym for REST as follows: **R**-Relinquish my expectations, **E**-Embrace the situation for what it is, **S**-Stop trying to control it and **T**-Trust God that He is actively working things out! Once I take the time to go through these steps of R.E.S.T, then I find that reflection easily follows.

# EACH DAY ANEW

Two dictionary definitions of *reflection* are "serious thought or consideration" and "an idea about something, especially one that is written down or expressed." I've discovered that times of rest and reflection can release creative thinking about life. This is the time to have a journal handy and "just start writing." Creative writing has no limits, it is simply allowing the activity of writing or typing to be an extension of your thoughts.

Two of my creative writing journal entries involve jigsaw puzzles and pianos.

IT'S PUZZLING . . . Life seems to get faster and faster. It's neat, though, to pause and see how the pieces of my life are beginning to fit together, like a million-piece jig-saw puzzle. It all looks impossible when you start but small areas at a time get filled in and before long the big picture is revealed.

I usually begin with the edge pieces which can be likened to a general plan or goal. Then my time and energy, along with people and circumstances, may dictate which areas of the overall puzzle I work on. Sometimes I focus on one piece of the puzzle and search for where it fits. At other times I look and look for what I think the puzzle piece should look like, only to be surprised when I get close to completing the puzzle and discover the piece was there all along, just much different than I expected.

Isn't it interesting how a simple thing like a jig-saw puzzle is so similar to how things may happen in our lives? Just something neat to think about!

IN NEED OF A TUNE-UP? I'm feeling *out of tune* with God lately and it seems like things are not going as well as I hoped. It brings to mind how a piano can be *in tune* or *out of tune*. Now, when a piano is *in tune* it is ready from the start for something good to come out of it. A piano *out of tune* will just not measure up. No matter how skilled the pianist, each note will fall short of its intended sound, making it flat or sharp. The original music score written to be a beautiful melody becomes twisted and distorted because the piano isn't *in tune*.

So it is with life. I cannot always control the situations in my life or the people who come along to interact with me. But I can be in control of how I respond and react. I don't have to settle for flats or sharps or disharmony in my life. I can be *in tune,* but I cannot *tune* myself. It takes a *piano tuner* to *tune* me.

Likewise, I need the Holy Spirit to examine my heart, reveal my shortcomings and sin, and cleanse me from all unrighteousness. Then my life will be like a piano that is *in tune*. Only then will the sounds that come forth produce something wholesome and beautiful to hear, whether it is the simple tune of *Chopsticks* or the masterpiece of *Beethoven's Fifth Symphony*.

Take time to rest, reflect and look within. Reflection can help us begin to understand what is of true value in our lives. Then we can better choose how to use our time and energy according to that which is truly important and not merely react to what seems to be urgent. The less we try to control and manipulate our own lives and live with a spirit of surrender to God's will and way, the more we will experience what He created us to be and learn how

He wants us to live. Gloria Gaither, a true wordsmith and songwriter, penned the following, "We don't get free by struggling, we get free by surrendering."

In *Wholehearted Faith* by Rachel Held Evans, she states, "The enemy of faith is not doubt, it is certainty." Faith is refined and actually grows stronger when we don't have control over the outcome. Accepting God's control over time (even the giving of it) can lead to a sense of relinquishment and relaxation which can bring about comfort and peace. Approaching *each day anew* involves learning to be patient and content with periods of waiting you encounter in life. You may find it's worth the wait – I do every time!

*The LORD is good to those who wait for Him,*
*to the soul who seeks Him.*
*It is good that one should wait quietly*
*for the salvation of the LORD.*
*Lamentations 3:25-26*
*(English Standard Version)*

# CHAPTER EIGHT

## Look Up:
## For Rainbows and Silver Linings

*You'll never find a rainbow looking down.*
Charlie Chaplin

Are you one who looks for the proverbial silver linings amidst the dark clouds? Do you view difficult circumstances more as obstacles or opportunities? Would you consider yourself to be easily discouraged or stubbornly persistent? No matter how we answer these questions, there may come seasons in each of our lives when we feel dismayed, stuck, or trapped. We might become haunted by our past, or we get frustrated with our present, or we can get caught up worrying about our future until we become anxious, disillusioned, and miserable. We then find ourselves trying every means possible to fix it, to get unstuck, to bring back meaning, motivation, and hope, but with little success.

During my seasons of discontent, I would find myself saying "What's wrong with me? I'm usually an optimistic and energetic person with my life organized and under control. Get a grip and get over it!" When life becomes overwhelming, we often try to regain control by working harder, by trying to reason ourselves through it, or figure out what needs changing and change it. But no matter how much I tried, I would sink deeper into what I can best describe as quicksand, or what David described in one of his Psalms as *a slimy pit of mud and mire*:

> I waited patiently for the LORD; He turned to me and heard my cry. He lifted me out of the slimy pit, out of the mud and mire; He set my feet on a rock and gave me a firm place to stand.
> (*Psalm 40:1-2, NIV*)

In my previous chapter, the emphasis was on taking time alone to rest, reflect and *look within*. These are tools that have helped me recognize my problems, my feelings, and how many of my self-efforts were futile in helping make things better.

However, it is important to distinguish that time spent alone can be different than the time we spend *alone with God*. This distinction in my journal entries may have become obvious by now. Taking time alone with God to reflect and write were instrumental in the inspiration I received as I contemplated what "rest" has meant for me. For purposes of review, my acronym for R.E.S.T. is **R**-Relinquish my expectations, **E**-Embrace the situation for what it is, **S**-Stop trying to control it and **T**-Trust God that He is actively working things out!

Spending time alone with God is an avenue for both learning and accepting His will. Of course, God knows and will act according to what is best for us, but we are still responsible for our own decisions and actions. Even if we find ourselves stuck, trapped, or in a miry pit as a consequence of following our own way (or due to other reasons), God is able to use any circumstance for our betterment and for the fulfillment of His good plan for our lives.

A verse from Jeremiah, a prophet from the Old Testament in the Bible, is one that brings hope in the midst of dire circumstances for God's people; both for Israel while exiled in Babylon as well as for us today. To get a fuller understanding of the encouraging words from Jeremiah 29:11, let's look at it in two translations and a paraphrase:

> For I know the plans I have for you, declares the LORD, plans to prosper you and not to harm you, plans to give you hope and a future.
> *(New International Version)*

> For I know the plans and thoughts that I have for you, says the LORD; plans for peace and well-being and not for disaster, to give you a future and a hope.
> *(The Amplified Version)*

> I know what I'm doing. I have it all planned out—plans to take care of you, not abandon you; plans to give you the future you hope for. *(The Message)*

Time with God and in His Word can also bring conviction of our own shortcomings and sin, as well as discovery of changes we need make in order to act upon how He is leading. Conviction may not be pleasant, but it has its rewards. Conviction, commitment, and motivation may be sequentially related and have an impact on how we view our past, our present and even our future. Conviction can also be a point at which we become motivated to start *each day anew.*

Regardless of how we may become stuck, discouraged, disillusioned, or depressed, God knows and cares. He does not abandon us, and He will give us peace, well-being, and a hopeful future. God can also use the difficult circumstances in our lives to teach us more about *contentment.*

"Bloom where you are planted" is a very familiar saying that actually carries some truth. Perhaps we aren't as trapped in our difficult circumstances as we think if we view our current situation not as being trapped, but as one in which we are planted. But life isn't always about blooming. As gardeners know, often plants need pruning. Cutting back of all that is unhealthy or dead actually provides an opportunity for greater growth and productivity to occur.

Winter is an important season, in the plant world as well as in our own lives. During the dormant stage in the plant world, growth, development, and physical activity are temporarily stopped, minimizing metabolic activity, and helping conserve energy for future periods of growth and vitality.

The Apostle Paul tells us that there is indeed growth that comes from our periods of longsuffering:
> ...but we rejoice in our sufferings, knowing that suffering produces endurance, and endurance produces character, and character produces hope (*Romans 5:3-4, ESV*)

Eleanor Roosevelt, a woman of great faith and character, has a quote that speaks to me about endurance in the midst of the dormant periods of our lives. She states, *"In the midst of Winter, I discover within myself an invincible Summer."* Invincible can be defined as *too powerful to be overcome*. This definition certainly doesn't refer to anything that resides in me alone, especially when I am going through a season of dormancy, discouragement, or depression. No, the power that resides in me to keep on keeping on, to walk by faith and not by sight, to look for that silver lining in the clouds of despair and to know that the promise of a rainbow is only fulfilled following a storm, <u>comes from God</u>!

Another special inspiration of mine has been my very dear cousin, Suzanne. Uncle Sam, who initially inspired me to write, was her father. Like Uncle Sam, Suzanne is also quite an amazing and unforgettable character. She is the type of person who attacks life with a vitality and a vigor that even makes my head spin. She is adventurous and courageous and loves people and places and life, simply because people and places and life are meant to be loved.

In spite of her love of adventure, Suzanne still recognizes the truth that underlies true contentment in life. She would tell you in a minute that it's not trips around the world, or money, or education that give daily life its meaning, instead it's special moments along the way that count, such as sharing a smile with a stranger, spending time with a loved one, standing in awe of God's handiwork in nature, or merely being alone - and still - and knowing that God is with us and always will be. Suzanne wrote the following poem over 40 years ago which expresses these sentiments.

STAND STILL, LOOK UP, LOOK BEYOND

*Stand still.*
Stand still for a moment,
Stop for a bit amidst empty laughter,
                shattered dreams,
                endless aggravation and
*Stand still.*

*Look up.*
Look up to the sky,
Look beyond the scurrying,
        frowns,
        emptiness,
        congestion surrounding,
              drowning,
                  threatening you and
*Look up.*

The sky is our refuge.
It is forever constant,
        all-seeing, offering
              the warmth of the sun,
              the wonder of the stars,
              the delight of the clouds

The eagle knows the wisdom of the sky.
He pauses only briefly among those
        who haven't discovered
        the comfort, the freedom,
        the undemanding place
Where he calls his home.

The flower knows the majesty of the sky.
She lives each day gazing in awe
        at her canopy,
        her shelter,
        her kind protector.
She does not seem to see
        the rushing, stomping,
        careless creatures
        towering above her, but
*Looks beyond.*

> I cannot soar with the wings of a bird,
> I do not have roots like the flower,
> > anchoring me to the earth,
> But I was given a soul
> > to experience,
> > to comprehend,
> > to worship God,
> To *Stand Still*,
> To *Look Up*,
> To *Look Beyond!*
>
> R. Suzanne Cochran.
> March 4, 1976.

If you really think about it, our lives are very insignificant and short compared to eternity and God's master plan of the universe. Yet, God loves us enough to make our lives have worth and meaning and each moment can be so precious if we'll only rely on God and have faith in the fact that He will supply our needs and direct our paths. Taking time to shift my focus off myself and more onto how God is at work in my life and the lives of others causes me to shift my attitude toward praise and gratitude. It even causes me to focus on praising and thanking others more.

How often do we pause for a moment to give praise or thanks to someone? One simple affirmation or a word of thanks can make such a difference in the lives of those around us. How much more important it is to take time to praise our Creator and Heavenly Father for *Who* He is and thank Him for *What* He has done! Reflecting upon *Who* God is and *What* He has done inspired me to compose several poems. These are written *to God* and are an attempt to praise Him and in some small way communicate my love and appreciation for what He has done in my life and what He continues to do daily.

### PRAISE BE TO GOD

Praise be to God, my strength and my hope,
He saves me when I'm at the end of my rope.
He shares in my joy and He eases my sorrow,
He gives me a reason for facing tomorrow.
I sing to Him, talk to Him, walk with Him, love Him,
In all of the world there is no one above Him.
As my Father, I respect Him and believe He can't falter,
It's exciting to know I'm His very own daughter!

"PRAISE BE TO THE LORD" is my jubilant cry,
For my soul is the Lord's, even though my body die.

### HE

He who amazes,
Who raises,
Who dazes,
This Almighty One
Let us praise and adore.
Amen.

### THANKS, GOD

I want to say "thank you"
But words can't convey
These very deep feelings
That I send your way.

So, when I say "thank you"
I want you to know
My feelings are greater than
My words can show.

Sometimes it is hard
To know how to start,
So, thank you, Dear Lord,
For hearing my heart!

At other times, my writing took a different direction in affirming God for His direction and guidance in my life.

## MORNING, NOON OR NIGHT

Morning, Noon, or Night,
When there is darkness, He's my light.
When things are blurry, He's my sight.
He makes the wrong things turn out right.
My God, He's really out-a-sight!
But that-'s alright,
Cause I know He's real, and that's how I feel.

## DEAR FATHER

Dear Father, hear me as I pray,
Please help me through tomorrow's day.

A test at nine, please clear my mind,
And help me think things logically.
Then papers due, and speech class too,
Another test awaits at three.

It's really nice to know You're near
And that these things You seek to hear.
Now I can rest my weary head
Knowing tomorrow presents no dread.

So, when tomorrow's day comes due
I hope and pray, for Thee I may
Live not for me, but YOU.

## SHINE, MY LIGHTHOUSE

Shine, my lighthouse, strong and clear,
Guide me through my doubts and fears.
Lead me on through higher seas,
To do Thy will, My God to please!

Shine, my lighthouse, let me know
With certain signals, where to go.
Without your guidance I would be
A forlorn sailor lost at sea,
Not knowing what life held for me.

So, Shine, my lighthouse,
Shine for me!

Praise and thanksgiving can dispel discouragement and have certainly been instrumental in helping me start *each day anew*! Whatever time you give to *be still*, to *look beyond* your current feelings and circumstances and *look up* to God is really time well invested. In Matthew 6:6 we find, "Go into your closet, shut the door, pray to the Father, and He who sees you will reward you openly." God has indeed rewarded me and continues to reward me daily, in tangible and intangible ways that I call blessings. You, too, can receive blessings beyond all you can imagine. All it takes is a little giving on your part; of yourself, your own will, and an intentional effort to *take time*. Is that too much to ask? You decide.

> ***Therefore, we do not lose heart.***
> ***Though outwardly we are wasting away,***
> ***yet inwardly we are being***
> ***renewed day by day.***
> ***For our light and momentary troubles***
> ***are achieving for us an eternal glory***
> ***that far outweighs them all.***
> ***So, we fix our eyes not on what is seen,***
> ***but on what is unseen,***
> ***since what is seen is temporary,***
> ***but what is unseen is eternal.***
> ***2 Corinthians 4: 16-18***
> ***(English Standard Version)***

# CHAPTER NINE

## Give It All You've Got And Go for It!

*"Let us not pray to be sheltered from dangers but to be fearless in facing them..."*
Tagore, *Fruit Gathering*

As I write this chapter, the 24th Winter Olympics are occurring. I am a fan of the Olympics, both Winter and Summer games. I have my favorite events that I follow, but I do tune into other events as well. I like to hear the background stories of the competitors and then follow their efforts and outcomes in their events. It means so much more than just seeing the top three medalists standing on podiums while flags are raised, and an anthem played. The athletes each have been on a journey and through a grueling and tedious process, often over many years leading up to being selected as a part of the elite team of Olympic competitors.

This year there have been several competitors in their mid-30's, some having competed in up to four previous Olympics. This impresses me for several reasons. First, their commitment over a prolonged period of time, in this case over twenty years since most Olympic athletes begin their journey and training as children. Secondly, they are competing against other athletes half their age and often face criticism that they are beyond their prime. But most of all, it inspires me that they still "give it all they've got and go for it," even when it involves life-threatening feats such as racing up to eighty miles an hour down slippery slopes in the downhill skiing event or twisting around in breathtaking contortions mid-air, hoping to land in just the right way in the various alpine events.

When interviewed, one of these older athletes mentioned the privilege it had been just to be a part of the history and development of their sport. They commented how some of the younger teammates had shared with them how they had been inspired as children watching them compete in those earlier Olympic contests. One Olympic competitor even gave her place to compete in an event to another team member who ended up making history! What a legacy to leave! Inspiring others' lives goes way beyond standing on an Olympic podium or even breaking a world record. At a time in our world where people are more likely to look out for themselves first, this kind of self-sacrifice speaks mightily.

Another inspiration I receive from the Olympic athletes is watching how they handle themselves when they finish their event after not doing as well as they had hoped. Those who take it in stride remind me of the concept that it is not so much what happens to you that is all important, rather it is how you handle what happens to you that really helps you grow better, not bitter. Even though most of us are not Olympic-minded individuals, we can still learn how a persistent and positive attitude can be a very useful tool in helping us handle what happens to us.

Winston Churchill, Prime Minister of England during World War II, was a great leader and motivational speaker. One of his quotes stresses the importance of perseverance: *"Success is never final; failure is never fatal; it is the courage to continue that counts."*

A motto I can recall becoming so popular that it ended up on T-shirts, tea towels and signs, among other things, was "When life gives you lemons, make lemonade." As I contemplated this saying, I decided that, of course, a sweetener is needed to make good lemonade, and with my southern tastebuds, that would mean lots of sugar.

In applying this to real life, I considered that making lemonade from life's lemons would best include the sweetener of a persistent and positive attitude. A further Christian application would claim that the best lemonade we can make out of the lemons in our lives actually begins with the ingredient of the refreshing water that only God can provide, as Christ proclaims He is the Living Water!

Now an important fact to note is, that in reality, not all lemons have lemonade potential. Some are simply sour experiences that have to be endured and they can really (pardon the expression) "suck." Or perhaps with the lemon imagery, a more polite expression would be that they can cause us to "pucker." Many unhealthy habits and even tragic consequences have occurred in people's lives who were trying to escape reality and the pain it can bring. Some even decided life wasn't worth living.

So how can we maintain a healthy balance when facing reality that is unpleasant or difficult? Consider a rose garden. When your life's journey affords you the opportunity to enjoy something good, like stopping to smell the roses, there is always the possibility of pain involved, such as getting scratched by the thorns. In the book, *I Never Promised You a Rose Garden* by Hannah Green, a young girl, along with the help of her therapist, struggles to learn how to face reality. Dr. Fried, the therapist, expresses the wonderful privilege we have in life, even when reality may include hardship or pain:

> "Look here," Dr. Fried said. "I never promised you a rose garden. I never promised you perfect justice . . . and I never promised you peace or happiness. My help is so that you can be free to fight

for all these things. The only reality I offer is the challenge to accept it or not, at whatever level you are capable."

Life certainly offers no guarantees, but what it does offer is opportunities and challenges. Even rose gardens have their share of thorns. It is the opportunity to see and smell such objects of beauty that make the risks involved worthwhile. When we realize this, we can fight against the tendencies that tempt us to want to escape reality. Instead, we can face them and deal with them in spite of the difficulties.

Joni Eareckson Tada, another one of my faith heroes, has faced over five decades of life in a wheelchair after a diving accident that left her paralyzed when she was a teenager. Joni also fights daily with chronic pain that she experiences even though she has paralysis. If that hasn't been enough of a battle, Joni also survived breast cancer. But she didn't just survive, she thrived! Joni's attitude and outlook on life reveals her secret:

> "I'm finding out more and more that reaching an earthly destination is merely incidental. It is in trusting and obeying the Lord Jesus Christ in each mile of the journey right now that counts . . . and the journey is a drama of choices and changes for us all."

Certainly, both choices and changes can be challenging, and even difficult at times. Additionally, our self-image as well as our self-confidence can vary many times in our lives.

When we recognize and accept change in our lives, it can actually help us maintain a balance that promotes contentment, no matter what our circumstances may be. And the choices we make, especially the thoughts we think, can be keys in approaching *each day anew*.

A particular lesson on this subject comes from one of my favorite children's books, *The Little Engine That Could*. In spite of size, ability or what seemed like an insurmountable obstacle (the mountain it needed to climb), the Little Engine's attitude of "I think I can, I think I can" is what helped propel it to success. However, *beware of believing that all power resides in positive thinking*.

For example, picture yourself behind the wheel of an automobile. If you determine a direction you desire to go, turn the ignition key, and prepare to put the car in drive, then you are at least making an effort to get going. However, your positive intentions and actions alone won't get you anywhere unless there is fuel in the car that will enable you to proceed with your journey. And even though you have in mind where you want to go and how to get there, more often than not you may encounter delays, roadblocks, detours, and changes to your original plans.

So, in approaching life's daily journey, it is important to realize that in addition to having a positive attitude, your tank must have the necessary fuel to get you where you want to go. As a Christian, this fuel for my life is the presence and filling of God's Holy Spirit. When I surrendered complete control of my life over to God's will for my life then I began to approach life His way. His way is faith in Christ Who is THE Way, THE Truth, and THE Life *(John 14:6, ESV)*.

Although I received the Holy Spirit when I first trusted Jesus as my Savior, there are still many opportunities, day to day, moment by moment, to receive a "re-filling" of the Spirit. There is one baptism of the Holy Spirit but many fillings. When I continually surrender faith in myself and exercise faith in Christ it is then that I receive fuel for my life – The Holy Spirit!

Even when things seem to be going our way and we feel like we're on a natural high, it is still possible to experience burnout. Any continual stress, whether good or bad, can lead to strain in life. That's why it's important to maintain a balance and a clear perspective.

A poem that means the world to me talks about the necessity of "resting" but not "quitting." This poem speaks to me in an extra special way. It was a favorite of my father's and hung on his office wall until the day he died. When unpacking his things over a year later, I found the poem, the frame tattered, and the parchment yellowed with age. The words seemed to speak to me as if they were being spoken by Daddy himself. Daddy was always behind me one hundred percent of the way, no matter what. His sense of confidence and self-assurance instilled in me the determination and will to turn defeat into success. In just a few words, the following poem by Frank Stanton, expresses what often takes years to learn.

### DON'T QUIT

When things go wrong, as they sometimes will,
When the road you're trudging seems all up hill,
When the funds are low and debts are high,
And you want to smile, but you have to sigh,
When cares are pressing you down a bit,
Rest, if you must – but don't you quit.

Life is queer with its twists and turns,
As everyone of us sometimes learns,
And many a failure turns about,
When he might have won had he stuck it out.
Don't give up, though the pace seems slow,
You might succeed with another blow.

Often the goal is nearer than
It seems to a faint and faltering man.
Often the struggler has given up
When he might have captured the victor's cup,
And he learned too late, when night slipped down,
How close he was to the golden crown.

Success is failure turned inside out,
The silver tint to the clouds of doubt,
And you never can tell how close you are,
It may be near when it seems afar.

So, stick to the fight when you're hardest hit,
It's when things seem worst that you mustn't quit.

If you want the most out of life, you've got to give life the best you've got. Give it your all, even when your all may seem small. You cannot do all the good the world needs, but the world needs all the good you can do. Let go of your perceived limitations and trust God to work in you and through you for your good and His glory. The more you endeavor to trust God, the more He empowers you to do so. I have found that as I trust God, my daily journey often proves to be more meaningful than just reaching all the destinations on my to-do or to-go list.

Helen Keller, who was blind, deaf, and mute since birth, first learned how to communicate due to the persistence of her teacher, Annie Sullivan. Helen worked diligently all of her life and greatly inspired and encouraged many individuals that the world labeled handicapped. Helen expressed, *"I thank God for my handicaps, for through them I have found myself, my work and my God."* This attitude certainly embodies what Scripture tells us, that we are to "give thanks in all circumstances, for this is the will of God . . ." (I Thessalonians 5:18, ESV).

God also instructs us to seek, and we shall find; ask and it shall be given to us; knock and the door shall be opened. (Matthew 7:7, ESV). We are the ones who are instructed to do the seeking, the asking, and the knocking. Sometimes it may involve seeking different paths, asking different questions, and trying different doorknobs. What do you want out of life? What are you willing to risk? Give it all you've got and go for it! What may seem impossible for you, is possible with God. (*Luke 18:27, ESV*)

> **"And I am sure of this;
> that He Who began a good work in you
> will bring it to completion
> at the day of Jesus Christ."
> Philippians 1:6
> (English Standard Version)**

# CHAPTER TEN
## *The End?*

When writing a book, it's hard to know where to start and even more of a challenge to know when and how to end. My initial thought was that although this book is ending, our stories aren't. And this is true. But there seemed to be more that I wanted to say. Even though this book is coming to a close, my life's story still continues to be full of "new beginnings."

There is so much more to living than just reaching a destination. Meaning and enjoyment in life can be a part of our journey and not just a prize at the finish line. Granted, our earthly finish line is physical death. An entire philosophy has been built around "eat, drink and be merry, for tomorrow we die." However, if during our lives, we chase only what this world deems desirable, successful, or important, we will eventually become disappointed and disillusioned. We may even find ourselves miserable and cynical, living fearful and defeated lives.

Even though the world has many well-intentioned and good-hearted individuals, as well as worthwhile efforts, if we place our trust and value solely on what the world offers, we will rarely learn contentment, know the fullness of joy, experience lasting peace or find eternal hope. Contentment involves more than the body; it involves the soul and spirit. And a right relationship with God gives us guidance throughout our journey wherever it takes us.

Tragedies and traumas profoundly affect us, making contentment a challenge. However, when I approach my life with an attitude of gratitude, even though the pain and difficulties do not disappear, they do fade, and God's goodness prevails.

God's work during my childhood, with its many challenges, laid a firm foundation of His unfailing love, great faithfulness, and an awareness of His mercies new every morning. The loss of my earthly father when I was a teenager also directed my faith more toward dependence on my Heavenly Father and less on my earthly parents and any fleeting security they could provide.

My young adult years were spent pursuing the usual expectations such as college degrees, beginning a career, and discovering a relationship that would lead toward marriage. But also, I also experienced difficulties and detours in my life, with unexpected joint deterioration and replacement surgeries, losses of various kinds and painful emotional upheaval. The great challenge became one of living life "one day at a time," a lesson each of us must eventually learn.

I mentioned earlier how much my mother impacted my life and she continues to do so, even now, years after her life on earth ended. It is no coincidence that as I write these very words today, the calendar reminds me it is her birthday and I realize I'm wearing a favorite shirt of mine which belonged to her. Not long ago I took some time to reread some of Mother's writings that she left for us, simply entitled, "My Memories." Some excerpts really touched me, and I want to share some of them:

> My priority as a mother was to keep my family close and to instill in Candy that a "positive" attitude would see her through this illness. As parents, our goal was to give Rodney and Candy a loving and Christian home, and a good education. Based on this foundation, we could survive anything. This is not to say that we did not have many heartbreaking events during the following years, but God gave us faith and strength to cope each day. Candy underwent one life-threatening event, followed by many, many operations, but with good doctors and our faith in God, our close-knit family survived.
>
> I have so much for which to be thankful. It is so great to be at peace with God and have peace in my heart. Life has not been without turmoil, but I try to think positive thoughts and be happy. Positive thoughts, a smile to my neighbors and children (loved ones), and faith in the Good Lord are what bring me joy.

Mother was a survivor, from her birth as a three-pound premature baby not expected to live, until she took her final breath. Even though from outward appearances Mother weathered the challenges of aging with the grace of a genteel, southern lady, there were still difficult days when she would remind me repeatedly that "growing old ain't for sissies." However, her optimism would once again kick in and often, when asked how she was doing, her answer was "Well, I have been better, but I have been worse." Mother didn't just survive, she thrived.

Being able to share Mother's later years with her was truly a blessing as well as a challenge for both of us, as it involved Mother having to relinquish more and more of her ingrained and even hard fought-for independence. And I was the one she usually fought with.

Another one of Mother's sayings that I will forever hold in my heart is, "A son's a son 'til he takes a wife, but a daughter's a daughter all of her life." Mother would often repeat this when she was feeling particularly grateful for having me as a daughter. Thankfully, the battles lessened as time marched on. However, I would often hear Mother say, mainly in response to what she perceived as me telling her what to do, "I'll make my own decision, thank you." Even though her final days were spent peacefully resting, when I was giving her what I considered was permission to let go of this life and feel free to go on to heaven, I could still sense Mother communicating once again that "she would make her own decision, thank you."

After Mother's passing, Regina, one of Mother's regular daytime companions, sent me the following letter, full of precious memories about Mother:

> I will remember your mother's warm smile and graceful ways, our reading *The Daily Bread* devotion every day and never having a meal without saying grace. She would look at your picture and talk about how proud she was of her children and how attentive you were.
> She always reminded me how happy the entire family was when she was expecting your brother, knowing he would carry on the family name. She told me your real name was Candace, named by your grandmother, but your brother is the one who gave you the name Candy.
> She told about being an only child but never being lonely because she had cousins by the dozens always wanting to come stay overnight. Also, she said her grandmother lived with them for a while and her grandmother and her mother did all the cooking, and she was glad because she didn't like to cook but preferred to be outside with her daddy. She talked a lot about Aunt Prudie, her mother's baby sister, not much older than she was and more like a sister to her, educating her all about the facts of life. She loved spending time with her in Memphis every summer and how she would return with new clothes and shoes. She was especially proud that she was the first girl in her class to get a pair of high heel pumps.

> We talked often of Jackson, Mississippi. My mother was from Canton, and she knew where that was. She also talked a lot about "The Good Lord" and so did my mom who passed during the time I was helping your mother. Both their birthdays were in April. I felt especially close to your mother.

From three pounds to almost ninety-three years, Mother did more than survive – she confidently lived life to the fullest with a strong faith and dependence on the Good Lord – and blessed many along the way. In addition to Mother's written memories, we discovered words of wisdom written in her own handwriting, included with her final instructions:

> In times of stress and turmoil you have two options: you can collapse and give up or you can keep putting one foot in front of the other, look for the clouds to clear and eventually you will see your way out. Meanwhile, just focus on surviving with the help and hope God gives you."

I'm sure Mother's desire in sharing these wise words, as well as memories about her life, would be that whoever would read them would be encouraged to "keep on keeping on!" I know I have been greatly encouraged by her words and her life and continue to be challenged in the way I face life, each and every day. The impact of Mother's story continues beyond her earthly departure; an important legacy that lives on.

Much of Mother's life was spent putting another's needs before her own, demonstrating sacrificial love, just as her Savior and Lord, Jesus Christ did for her. As I write this final chapter, Good Friday is here with the celebration of Christ's resurrection and victory over death just days away. Jesus Himself spoke about self-sacrifice, as follows in the paraphrased version of Scripture, *The Message*:

> Self-sacrifice is the way, *My* way, to finding yourself, your true self. What good would it do to get everything you want and lose you, the real you? *(Luke 9:25)*

This reminds me of martyred missionary Jim Elliott's well-known quote, "He is no fool who gives what he cannot keep, to gain that which he cannot lose." Sacrificial giving and living mean "laying down of one's life." Near the end of His life, Jesus told his followers,

> This is my commandment, that you *love one another as I have loved you.* Greater love has no one than this, that a person will lay down his life for his friends." *(John 15:12-13, ESV)*

A person who embraces a caring lifestyle receives many blessings, whether or not the care is reciprocated. Another teaching of Jesus about giving is expressed well as follows:

> What I'm trying to do here is to get you to relax, to not be so preoccupied with *getting,* so you can respond to God's *giving.* People who don't know God and the way He works fuss over these things, but you know both God and how He works. Steep

your life in God-reality, God-initiative, God-provisions. Don't worry about missing out. You'll find all your everyday human concerns will be met. *(Matthew 6:33, The Message)*

As we grow in Christlikeness, serving others will become more a part of our lives. We do not need to be so self-consumed, for God takes care of our own needs, providing strength and refreshment when we have given our all in caring for others. I certainly found this to be true when caring for Mother as she aged, in addition to the challenges I faced in caring for my family.

If we place God at the center of our lives, embracing His truth, His ways, and His beauty, we will become stable, grateful, and satisfied – a great description of contentment. Working to maintain a proper balance of our emotions, especially overcoming negative emotions, is a big part of contentment.

Spending time alone with God and His Word is the main avenue for both learning and accepting His will, which can often differ from our own. Patience is key to waiting upon God to help us process our thoughts and feelings about the past, present and future. Accepting God's control and timing can actually lead to a sense of relief and relaxation which can bring comfort and peace.

If my heart could speak to you now, it would echo what the Apostle Paul exclaims, "Give thanks in all circumstances, for this is the will of God in Christ Jesus for you."*(1 Thessalonians 5:8, ESV)*. When you look closely at this verse, you see that we are to give thanks IN all circumstances, not FOR all circumstances.

We can better cultivate an attitude of gratitude when we also understand that "We can know that for those who love God all things work together for good, for those who are called according to His purpose." *(Romans 8:28, ESV)*
**My life is evidence of these truths.**

Even in the midst of the many storms in life, a relationship with Jesus Christ will sustain us and give us strength to endure and peace within. I praise God for what He has done for me and for what He continues to do in my life daily. WITHOUT HIM each day would simply be a dead end, full of continual doubt and worry and discouragement. The real joy is that WITH HIM we can have direction, we can have purpose and most importantly, we can start *each day anew*!

> **Let the peace of Christ rule in your hearts...**
> **Let the message of Christ**
> **dwell in you richly...**
> **And whatever you do,**
> **whether in word or deed,**
> **do it all in the name of the Lord Jesus,**
> **giving thanks to God the Father through Him.**
> **Colossians 3:15-17**
> **(English Standard Version)**

# ACKNOWLEDGEMENTS

Since it has taken me over 40 years to complete this project, the people who have been a part of my writing journey would comprise a list too extensive to name. However, in addition to ongoing encouragement from my family and friends, several persons do merit specific mention.

As I reflect on my early inspiration to write for others to read, I'm grateful for my junior high school English teacher, Mrs. Graham, who encouraged creative writing and sparked my initial interest in writing essays and poetry and entering writing contests. Later on, as a young adult who was eager to write a book, I'm so thankful for the very practical advice of my Uncle Sam, who challenged me to "just start writing."

Twenty years later, my life intersected with Karen, who became a dear friend as well as a very important motivator and writing mentor. She helped me understand the benefit of rewriting my manuscript to be more reader-based versus my original writer/journal-based style. Even though Karen moved away, her conceptual ideas and editorial notes guided my revision efforts over the next twenty years!

In 2020, when the pandemic halted outside activities that had filled many of my hours, I once again revisited the project of writing, and I committed to spend time regularly in an effort to revise and complete my book, *Each Day Anew*.

During this time, God brought into my life a wonderfully enthusiastic lady, Margaret, who had recently written and published her own book (*Permissible Pleasures*). Being likeminded, she became my much-needed writing coach. Margaret was always quick to cheer my successes in completing chapters and lovingly suggest changes that would enhance what I was trying to communicate. Another mutual friend, Betty, who had a good eye for grammar, spelling, and punctuation, became one of my initial editors. Of course, the final editorial privilege was reserved for my dear husband, Joel, whose opinion I value most of all!

When time came to begin the actual publishing process, I found Fiona Ferris' book, *The Chic Author,* to be invaluable. She gave both practical information, as well as a fantastic recommendation for a graphic artist. It was thrilling to see the book cover design become a reality, much thanks to Les of *germancreative* at fiverr.com. The cover photograph is a candid shot of me taken in a rose garden over 40 years ago by a photographer friend, Scott. The thoughts and emotions he captured that day have been a part of inspiring my dream of someday writing a book and using this photograph for its cover.

If you know me personally, then I consider our relationship to have been a part of my life's story and I'm grateful for whatever chapter or season of life we shared together.

Above all, I give glory and honor and wholehearted gratitude to our Creator God, my Heavenly Father; to His Son, my Savior and Lord, Jesus Christ; and to the Holy Spirit who indwells me, guides me, comforts me, and promises to never leave or forsake me. Without this Holy Trinity, my life's journey, both the process and the destination yet to come, would not have been filled with the purpose, meaning and hope of being able to approach *Each Day Anew*!

Blessings, Candy

*Indeed, it is in Him that we live and move and have our being.*
*Acts 17:28a*
*(J. B. Phillips New Testament)*

# A NOTE FROM THE AUTHOR

Wow! What a privilege it has been to share my story with you! The fact that *Each Day Anew* has been over 40 years in the making makes its completion a true celebration. Thank you for being a part of this celebration by choosing to read it!

My prayer is that *Each Day Anew* is more than an easy read or a way to get to know me better. I hope you will consider making time to rest, reflect and explore a personal relationship with our loving Creator God. If He is not already your Heavenly Father, I pray you will receive Jesus Christ as your Savior and Lord and join His wonderful and eternal family!

Your life story is equally important and worth sharing, even if just for your family. Journaling can become an avenue for you to identify or process your thoughts and feelings, and maybe write your own book!

I encourage and welcome comments, questions, and any part of your story you might be willing to share with me. My email is eachdayanew2022@craigtex.com. Also please do me the favor of leaving a review on Amazon or any of your other favorite social media.

*With Humble Gratitude, Candy*

# ABOUT THE AUTHOR

Candy Cochran Craig is a native Mississippian but has called Alabama home for over 30 years. She began writing as a young adult, mainly through journaling, and believes we all have stories to tell that will continue on, long after our earthly lives have ended.

Candy is married to her husband, Joel, who has faithfully loved and cared for her for over 38 years. God blessed them with an only, beloved son, Tony and more recently with a precious daughter-in-love, Megan. Gracie, their rescued Yorkipoo keeps them company now that they have an empty nest.

Both Candy and Joel are birdwatchers and like to travel. Candy's favorite books to read are mysteries, suspense, and biblical fiction. She also enjoys jigsaw puzzles and time spent with good friends. Candy has been involved in the *Moms in Prayer International* ministry for over 25 years and highly recommends prayer with other moms as an invaluable and eternal investment in the lives of our precious children and future generations. (For information about this ministry and how to get involved visit the website, momsinprayer.org).

Made in the USA
Columbia, SC
27 July 2022